Test-Taking Strategies for the
USMLE STEP 2 Exam:
Proven Methods to Succeed

Notice

Medicine is an ever-changing science. As new research and clinical experience broaden our knowledge, changes in treatment and drug therapy are required. The authors and the publisher of this work have checked with sources believed to be reliable in their efforts to provide information that is complete and generally in accord with the standards accepted at the time of publication. However, in view of the possibility of human error or changes in medical sciences, neither the authors nor the publisher nor any other party who has been involved in the preparation or publication of this work warrants that the information contained herein is in every respect accurate or complete, and they disclaim all responsibility for any errors or omissions or for the results obtained from use of the information contained in this work. Readers are encouraged to confirm the information contained herein with other sources. For example and in particular, readers are advised to check the product information sheet included in the package of each drug they plan to administer to be certain that the information contained in this work is accurate and that changes have not been made in the recommended dose or in the contraindications for administration. This recommendation is of particular importance in connection with new or infrequently used drugs.

Test-Taking Strategies for the
USMLE STEP 2 EXAM: Proven Methods to Succeed

Julia I. Reading

New York   Chicago   San Francisco   Athens   London   Madrid   Mexico City
Milan   New Delhi   Singapore   Sydney   Toronto

1 2 3 4 5 6 7 8 9 DSS 27 26 25 24 23 22

ISBN 978-1-264-25875-8
MHID 1-264-25875-5

The editors were Michael Weitz and Christina M. Thomas.
The production supervisor was Richard Ruzycka.
Project management was provided by Poonam Bisht, MPS Limited.
The cover designer was W2 Design.

Library of Congress Cataloging-in-Publication Data
Names: Reading, Julia I., author.
Title: Test-taking strategies for the USMLE step 2 exam : proven methods to succeed / Julia I. Reading.
Description: New York : McGraw Hill, [2023] | Includes bibliographical references and index. | Summary: "This text should serve to highlight test taking weaknesses and the skills or strategies that may be useful to improve those weaknesses. Such weaknesses include a poor approach to the exam, difficulty reasoning through concepts, difficulty categorizing information, and anchoring. These weaknesses are the focus of this text. There are also skills and strategies that are important to refine as we become expert test-takers, such as time management, approach to reviewing labs, dealing with under confidence, and re-viewing answer choices at the end of an exam. You will be lead through general and specific test taking skills and weaknesses with practice questions so that upon completion of this text, you will hopefully be fully equipped to achieve the score (and career) of your dreams"—Provided by publisher.
Identifiers: LCCN 2022014750 (print) | LCCN 2022014751 (ebook) | ISBN 9781264258758 (paperback) | ISBN 9781264258765 (ebook)
Subjects: MESH: Clinical Medicine | Test Taking Skills | Examination Questions
Classification: LCC RC58 (print) | LCC RC58 (ebook) | NLM WB 18.2 | DDC 616.0076—dc23/eng/20220609
LC record available at https://lccn.loc.gov/2022014750
LC ebook record available at https://lccn.loc.gov/2022014751

McGraw Hill books are available at special quantity discounts to use as premiums and sales promotions, or for use in corporate training programs. To contact a representative please visit the Contact Us pages at www.mhprofessional.com.

Dedicated to my father

Contents

Introduction

Has there ever been a time when your exam score did not seem to reflect your knowledge level? Or a friend who was less prepared than you but still scored higher?

This is likely a reflection of your test-taking skills.

In my experience, differences in academic performance are often attributed to intelligence, memorization abilities, or time dedicated to studying. But how much of these differences should be attributed to test-taking skills instead?

First, we need to answer the question, what are test-taking skills?

Almost any factor that influences your performance on a test, outside of your knowledge base, is a test-taking skill. More formally, test-taking skills can be defined as "cognitive skills that strongly affect students' performance in tests."[1]

Some test-taking skills are likely very well known to you, including confidence, anxiety management, and time management. Other test-taking skills are not as well recognized. Some examples include the ability to deal with difficult questions, apply fund of knowledge to different scenarios, appropriately categorize information, strategy for reviewing answers, and reasoning abilities.[1,2]

The research on the importance of test-taking skills is compelling. Studies have demonstrated that even students with a good knowledge base still do poorly on exams, largely or in part due to a lack of test-taking skills.[3] Inversely, students who are apt in test-taking skills have been found to better demonstrate their knowledge on exams.[4]

If test-taking skills are so important for performance and demonstration of knowledge, then one would think that these skills are taught readily medical school. But how much of your medical education was dedicated to honing these skills?

I would guess very little.

In my experience, while this concept is largely supported in the literature, test-taking skills are not commonly taught. I have often wondered whether this is because of a shared belief that test-taking skills can't be taught. But can't all skills be taught?

When we think about learning a new language, a new sport, or a new hobby, it is common sense that we need to learn both about the activity and the skills needed to apply our knowledge about that activity.

Consider the process of learning a new language. Imagine sitting through lectures about grammar and vocabulary without ever being taught how to string vocabulary words together into sentences to have a conversation. And just like learning a new language, a new sport, or a new hobby, we are not expected to be born with the skills we need to be successful.

The same should be true for test-taking skill instruction.

And in a field like medicine, where your career can be determined by a single score, teaching these skills should be a priority.

As a tutor in medical school, I had many students who recognized their poor test-taking skills as a weakness but had resigned themselves to the belief that poor test-taking was their destiny, an unshakable quality, and just something to try to overcome on their resume with other skills and extracurricular activities. On day one of teaching these students, I marketed my philosophy on test-taking skills, but I was often met with the same story. My students often felt that they were inherently "bad test-takers" and preferred to study content rather than do practice questions. Many said they preferred to save practice questions until they had a better grasp on the material. But if answering questions is half the battle on the exam, then why would you spend 100% of your time on content alone?

Most likely, this aversion to practicing test questions stemmed from lack of confidence and poor understanding about how to effectively learn from practice questions. And without an adequate study resource available, it's no wonder students focused on content over application and practice.

After warming up to my philosophy and scoring higher on their exams, my students shared their frustration that they had struggled so much in medical school, and even undergraduate school, without any available resources to help them overcome what they knew was already a weakness for them, only now to realize this was a weakness they could overcome.

Medical students need to receive adequate training to successfully utilize their fund of knowledge and excel on standardized exams. This training should be just as fundamental to education as are lectures on kidney and cardiac function. We cannot be expected to succeed with one and not the other.

While the importance of test-taking skills is well demonstrated in the literature, instruction on how to teach test-taking skills is lacking. A literature review done in 2017 by Guerrasio et al was unable to find any research on the subject.[5] And unsurprisingly, there is no mainstream resource that specifically addresses deficiencies in test-taking strategy.

If test-taking skills are so undertaught, why don't test writers design more straightforward exams?

The fact that medical board exams remain reliant on skills other than the ability to memorize facts suggests that test writers find something inherently valuable in the qualities that are demonstrated through good test-taking skills. And while I don't disagree, the problem is for those who are at an unfair disadvantage due to lack of lifelong teaching and/or practice.

Why would test writers value test-taking skills?

Just like being an excellent physician, an excellent test-taker must be able to identify a problem, quickly formulate differential diagnoses, categorize the information provided, and filter out unimportant information from that which is important. They need to use this information to alter the probabilities of those differentials that they have identified and then need to generate a conclusion and an action plan.

While some test-taking skills may translate to those skills of a physician, it would still be unreasonable to conclude that a poor test taker is destined to become a poor physician. In fact, numerous studies demonstrate the lack of correlation between standardized test scores and clinical performance.[6,7]

The fact is that every medical student should have the resources they need to succeed available to them. While I can't say for certain why test-taking skill teaching has lagged so profoundly, I can say that my mission is to help students feel empowered to change their standardized performance in a way that they may have never previously thought possible.

My disclaimer: In medicine, test-taking skills do not exist in isolation from the material. As said by Guerrasio et al 2014, far more eloquently, *"If both deficits exist, knowledge must be remediated first, to provide the foundation to develop clinical reasoning skills."*[8] Keeping in mind that there is no way that we can know everything about medicine, test-taking skills will help us to arrive at the best answer even when we do have gaps in knowledge.

This text should serve to highlight your test-taking weaknesses and the skills or strategies that may be useful to you. After combining my years of teaching with the available literature, I have identified what I believe are the main test-taking weaknesses. These include a nonstrategic approach, difficulty reasoning through concepts and categorizing information, and anchoring bias. These weaknesses will be the focus of this text. We will also review skills and strategies that are important to refine as we become expert test-takers, such as time management, approach to reviewing labs, dealing with underconfidence, and reviewing answer choices at the end of an exam.

I will lead you through general and specific test-taking skills and weaknesses with practice questions. You will find that single questions are analyzed in depth over many, many pages. While this may seem excessive, I recommend devoting this time early on to develop your skills. The more you practice test-taking skills, the more implicit these will become, and the closer you will be to attaining the score (and career) of your dreams.

REFERENCES

1. Dodeen, H. (2009). Test-Related Characteristics of UAEU Students: Test-Anxiety, Test-Taking Skills, Guessing, Attitudes toward Tests, and Cheating. *Journal of Faculty of Education* (26), 31–66.
2. McLellan, J., & Craig, C. (1989). *Facing the Reality of Achievement Tests.* Education Canada (29), 36–40.
3. Vattanapath, R., & Jaiprayoon, K. (1999). An assessment of the effectiveness of teaching test-taking strategies for multiple-choice English reading comprehension tests. *Occasional Papers*, 8, 57–71.
4. Yun Peng, Eunsook Hong & Elsa Mason (2014). Motivational and cognitive test-taking strategies and their influence on test performance in mathematics. *Educational Research and Evaluation*, 20(5), 366–385, doi:10.1080/13803611.2014.966115.
5. Guerrasio, J., Nogar, C., Rustici, M., Lay, C., & Corral, J. (2017). Study Skills and Test Taking Strategies for Coaching Medical Learners Based on Identified Areas of Struggle. *MedEdPORTAL*, 13. doi:10.15766/mep_2374-8265.10593.
6. Campos-Outcalt, D., Rutala, P. J., Witzke, D. B., & Fulginiti, J. V. (1994). Performances of underrepresented-minority students at the University of Arizona College of Medicine, 1987–1991. *Acad Med*, 69(7), 577–582. doi:10.1097/00001888-199407000-00015.
7. Silver, B., & Hodgson, C. S. (1997). Evaluating GPAs and MCAT scores as predictors of NBME I and clerkship performances based on students' data from one undergraduate institution. *Acad Med*, 72(5), 394–396. doi:10.1097/00001888-199705000-00022.
8. Guerrasio, J., Garrity, M. J., & Aagaard, E.M. (2014). Learner deficits and academic outcomes of medical students, residents, fellows, and attending physicians referred to a remediation program, 2006–2012. *Acad Med.* 89(2):352–358. doi:10.1097/ACM.0000000000000122. PMID: 24362382.

1

Skills & Pitfalls

■ SECTION 1: TIMING

Why is it that some people finish an exam early, while others can't even get through all the questions in the allotted time frame?

Consider the following scenario. Student A reads each sentence of the vignette in great detail. They highlight each and every piece of information, including every symptom and physical exam finding.

How would you describe Student A's approach?

Student A is assigning equal energy and time to each sentence in the vignette as they search for clues that point to an answer. While this may not be the most time-efficient approach, Student A believes this approach will help to ensure that no information is missed.

But just because we read every word of every sentence doesn't mean we understand the relevance or the significance. We need to have a strategy.

Student A is not using any specific strategy, but still hopes to arrive at the correct answer. This approach might work for straightforward questions, but it will prove less useful for questions that require application of knowledge and problem solving.

Not only is this approach unadvisable from a strategy perspective, but it requires more time and energy. In my experience, this time and energy expenditure does not translate into better results.

The key is to use an approach that will increase your probability of answering the question correctly while also maximizing your time and energy efficiency on exam day.

Should student A read every word of the vignette with the same energy?

Student A should devote disproportionate energy to those aspects of the vignette that will lead them to the correct answer through practice and pattern recognition. They should learn how to avoid wasting time on those aspects that are redundant or misleading.

Many, if not all, of the test-taking skills described in this text should provide you with skills to generate a road map for each vignette. This road map should help to determine how to allocate a disproportionate amount of attention and energy towards certain parts of the vignette while neglecting others.

As your skills develop, you may even find that you can arrive at the correct answer after only reading a portion of the vignette.

This may seem counterintuitive.

Shouldn't *not* reading the entire vignette reduce your chances of scoring higher?

There is a fine balance between reading too much and too little of a vignette. On one hand, reading too much may predispose to certain pitfalls like second guessing, while reading too little may predispose to missing key information.

The USMLE Step 2 Exam is approximately nine hours long. You need enough time to answer all those questions and perform just as well on the first section as the last. Both time and energy are important factors, and the more you waste, the less you have.

If done correctly, you can learn to read and attend to only the important pieces of information and ignore the unimportant parts of the vignette. With time, you can develop the confidence to stop reading and move on once you have arrived at the correct answer.

The goal is to read smarter, not more.

Let's return to the scenario with student A.

After spending time ruminating over the answer choices, student A is still unsure of the answer, despite having read the vignette slowly and thoughtfully. Student A had hoped that they could figure out the answer if they devoted enough time to the problem.

What do you think the chances are that Student A will select the correct answer?

Consider the Law of Diminishing Returns to answer this question.

Energy devoted to the first 1 to 2 minutes on a question are highly productive. Chances of selecting the correct answer during this time period are high. Let's imagine that the success rate is 80% if done within the first 2 minutes.

At minutes 2 through 4, that same amount of energy becomes less productive. If you did not answer the question within the first 2 minutes, let's imagine the chances you answer the question correctly are now 40%. This represents the Law of Diminishing Returns. At a certain point, that energy will be better spent on a different question where there is still a high return rate.

After 4 minutes, that same amount of energy is even less productive, or possibly even counterproductive. Let's imagine the likelihood that you answer this question correctly is less than 20%. And at this point, you are allocating precious time and energy to a question that you are unlikely to answer correctly. To make matters worse, the chances of answering other questions correctly may fall as you start to feel more rushed. Your confidence may start to plummet. This represents the Law of Negative Returns.

Based on the Laws of Diminishing and Negative Returns, disproportionate allocation of time and energy to questions that can be answered more quickly should increase the chances of a higher exam score. Why spend an extra 3 to 5 minutes dissecting those challenging questions in hopes of arriving at the correct answer when those extra minutes would be far more useful on a question that you are more likely to answer correctly? Instead, use whatever time is leftover at the end of the exam to try and figure out the answers to the more difficult questions.

This strategy is especially useful for those students who tend to run out of time towards the end of the exam.

How many times have you run out of time, only to have to randomly guess on the last five questions?

Imagine this scenario for Student B. They run out of time at the end of their exam and are forced to guess on the last five questions. These questions would have been easy for Student B to answer correctly, had they had the time to read through them. They ran out of time because of some harder questions earlier on in the exam that they spent time thinking about. But even with that effort, Student B is not sure that they answered them correctly.

In this scenario, they were unlikely to answer those last five questions correctly through guesswork. They were also less likely to answer those harder questions earlier on in the exam correctly. This means that Student B was unlikely to answer ten questions correctly.

Imagine instead that Student B triaged their questions and allocated more time to those questions that they were more likely to answer correctly, leaving the five most challenging questions to answer last. The chance of answering these questions correctly was already low. If they still had run out of time, and had to guess on these last five questions, the result would not differ significantly. Now, Student B was unlikely to answer five questions correctly, rather than ten.

This second scenario is more likely to result in a higher score for Student B. Running out of time in the second scenario had a lesser effect on their score than in the first scenario.

These scenarios should demonstrate the importance of allocating time disproportionately in favor of those questions that you are more likely to answer correctly.

If there is spare time at the end of an exam, then you can run out the clock attempting to overcome the odds of choosing the wrong answer on those tougher questions. And if there isn't spare time, then there may not be a big difference in your score regardless.

This recommendation is contrary to the more common piece of advice to allocate the same amount of time for each question.

But does it truly make sense to allocate the same amount of time to each question?

All questions are not created equal. And while intuitively it makes sense to devote more time to those harder questions, it makes more sense probabilistically to do the opposite.

SUMMARY

1. Utilize strategies that prevent aimless and undirected reading. Read instead with a plan in mind.
2. Allocate differential energy to those parts of the vignette that are most relevant.
3. Avoid ruminating over answer choices.
4. The more time you spend on a question, the less likely you are to answer it correctly. This is the Law of Diminishing Returns.
5. Spend the most amount of time on questions that you are most likely to answer correctly.
6. Any extra time can be used to work through the more challenging questions.

■ SECTION 2: REVIEWING LAB VALUES

You will hear conflicting advice about whether to read labs before or after the vignette. There is no one right answer. But my preference is to review labs before reading the vignette.

Labs provide key insight into the pathophysiology of the scenario and as such will significantly alter your differential diagnoses. They should shape your expectations and shift your attention to what is most relevant. Because of this, you won't have to work as hard to dissect the vignette if you have first read the labs.

Reading the labs ahead of time allows you to develop a hypothesis unobstructed by clinical clues. This can protect you against traps set by the test writer.

In fact, after reading the labs, the question, and the answer choices, there is likely to be a high probability that you can answer the question correctly without even reading the vignette. This means that, by the time you arrive at the vignette, any extra information you encounter will either serve to support or dissuade the conclusions you have already made.

Labs can also be more straightforward than clinical clues described in a vignette. While a low hemoglobin always represents anemia, fatigue or pallor can be caused by any number of etiologies. And there are only so many variations to lab values on standardized exams.

So, I recommend reading the labs first, and using them as a guide for when you begin reading the vignette.

This brings up the question of how to review labs.

You know you need to pay attention to abnormal lab values. But the absence of certain abnormal labs (or findings) can be equally important, and you should practice noting those "pertinent negatives." As you build your knowledge base, you will have a better sense of the pertinent negatives for each clinical scenario to shape your differential diagnoses.

And, just like your approach to questions, your approach to interpretation of labs should have some sort of structure.

The items measured, regardless of whether there are abnormalities present or absent, can already begin to shape your differential diagnoses. For example, if thyroid studies were done, regardless of if they were negative, your differential should include diagnoses that may have overlap in signs or symptoms with thyroid disease.

If only one lab is abnormal, then the diagnosis is often clear. But in the case of many lab abnormalities, results become much harder to interpret.

The presence of multiple lab abnormalities requires you to understand pathophysiology a little more. Reasoning becomes hugely important in these cases. Reasoning is discussed in detail in Chapter 3.

Illness scripts should also make it easier to come up with a diagnosis from a constellation of abnormal lab values.

What is an illness script?

Put simply, an illness script is a mental summary or representation of a disease. This will be discussed in more detail in Chapter 4. The more you can develop your illness scripts, the more quickly you will be able to interpret labs and arrive at the correct diagnosis.

In terms of reviewing specific lab studies, let's begin with the Complete Blood Count (CBC).

How should we review a CBC?

We should first evaluate whether our patient has anemia or polycythemia. We can do so by reviewing the hemoglobin and hematocrit levels. Anemia will be far more common than polycythemia.

Polycythemia only has a few causes. The most common causes on board exams are from a genetic mutation, volume contraction, or secondary to increased erythropoietin (EPO) production. Increased EPO production can occur as a response to chronically decreased oxygen availability or from EPO producing tumors.

If we see an isolated polycythemia, we might suspect an EPO producing tumor. But, if we see signs of alkalosis and sodium derangements, we might suspect dehydration.

Polycythemia is not a highly tested concept. As often mentioned, highly tested concepts on board exams tend to be those conditions that are dangerous, common, or have complicated and/or easily testable pathophysiology. Polycythemia does not meet these criteria.

In contrast, anemia is a heavily tested concept. First, anemia is a very common condition. Second, identification of the etiology of anemia can be highly complicated and requires knowledge of underlying pathophysiology. Third, anemia can be dangerous in acute and/or severe settings. The criteria for a high yield concept in this case have been met.

If anemia is identified with either the hematocrit or hemoglobin, you should first evaluate whether this is a macrocytic, normocytic, or microcytic anemia. You can do so with the mean corpuscular volume (MCV) (Figure 1-1).

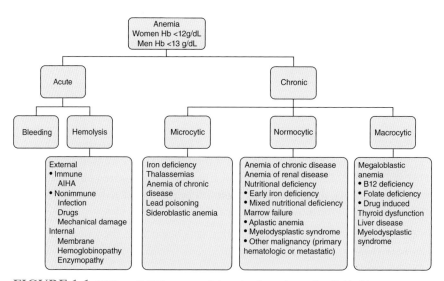

FIGURE 1-1 **Differential Diagnoses of Anemia**. Anemia can be divided into macrocytic, microcytic, and normocytic based on MCV. Acute anemia from bleeding or hemolysis will present as a normocytic anemia. (Reproduced with permission from McKean SC, Ross JJ, Dressler DD, Scheurer DB. *Principles and Practice of Hospital Medicine*, 2nd ed. McGraw Hill, 2017.)

What are common causes of macrocytic anemia?

Macrocytic anemia typically represents a folate or B12 deficiency. Less commonly tested on board exams, macrocytic anemia can also result from liver failure.

How can we use our knowledge of pathophysiology to help us differentiate between B12 or folate deficiency?

Like any vitamin deficiency, folate and B12 deficiencies can result from poor diet. Sometimes a deficiency may arise due to a medication side effect. Because B12 stores take several years to deplete, folate deficiency is more commonly the correct answer. But not always.

How else can we differentiate folate and B12 deficiencies?

Folate is an essential building block for DNA replication. In the case of medications that interfere with DNA replication, hematologic malignancies with cell overproduction, or pregnancy, folate is rapidly depleted.

B12 deficiency leads to an increase in methylmalonic acid. In the case of B12 deficiencies, buildup of methylmalonic acid will result in neurologic symptoms in the presence of macrocytic anemia.

After identifying a macrocytic anemia on exam, we will typically need to use clues from the vignette to finalize our diagnosis.

In contrast to macrocytic anemia, normocytic anemia is highly common in the population and high yield for exams.

Can you think of some causes of normocytic anemia?

We can divide normocytic anemia into two categories: Underproduction or destruction.

The most common causes of underproduction anemias are from hematologic malignancy or early iron deficiency. On the other hand, destruction anemias are caused by hemolysis. Hemolysis is most often autoimmune, but it can be caused by shearing forces from structures such as microthrombi on the walls of the vasculature or mechanical valves.

We can use the reticulocyte count to help distinguish between underproduction or destruction normocytic anemia.

A high reticulocyte count suggests there is destruction of red blood cells. The bone marrow is trying to compensate for increased destruction by producing more red blood cells than usual.

In the case of anemia, is a reticulocyte count of 1–3% normal?

The lab value key will tell you that a reticulocyte count of 1–3% is normal.

But if we are anemic, we should expect an increase in red blood cell production to compensate. A count of 1–3% is inappropriate and suggests an underproduction anemia. Something is preventing the bone marrow from increasing red blood cell production.

Why are anemias of destruction or underproduction normocytic, rather than micro- or macrocytic?

In anemias of underproduction or destruction, the problem is with a failure to initiate red blood cell synthesis or with destruction of red blood cells once they are synthesized.

Microcytic and macrocytic anemias are a result of a problem at some point in the red blood cell synthesis pathway resulting in an abnormally large or small red blood cell.

Microcytic anemias result from a problem with one of the major components of a red blood cell: Globin or heme. Heme is made up of iron and a porphyrin ring. If there are insufficient amounts of any of these components, then the red blood cell will undergo an additional cell division to increase the hemoglobin concentration in a particular cell.

The details and distinctions of the microcytic anemias are heavily tested on Step 1. But on Step 2, the focus is more clinical. This is where we can keep our focus.

Macrocytic anemias result from a problem with DNA building blocks. In the process of red blood cell division, there are insufficient DNA building blocks to complete the typical number of cellular divisions, resulting in a larger than usual red blood cell.

Interpretation of other isolated CBC abnormalities tends to be more straighforward.

When there are multiple abnormalities, such as pancytopenia, the most common causes include medication side effects, autoimmune conditions, or hematologic malignancies.

Let's move on to the Basic Metabolic Panel.

What is the best way to review a Basic Metabolic Panel?

A good place to start is by assessing fluid status.

To assess fluid status, we should have a strong understanding of basic pathophysiology and how this will represent itself in labs. Understanding this pathophysiology well will enable us to reason through almost any question with related lab values.

Let's begin by discussing sodium in the context of fluid status.

Sodium will be the best indicator for dehydration. You can see both hyper- and hyponatremia in the case of dehydration.

Hypernatremia is one of the more straightforward findings and most often indicates dehydration.

Why does hypernatremia indicate dehydration?

Consider this problem like a glass of water. Loss of water with the same amount of sodium will result in a more concentrated solution and an elevated sodium.

But why do you also see hyponatremia in the setting of dehydration?

Once your volume is *very* depleted, ADH no longer functions as normal to regulate sodium. Instead, ADH is recruited to reabsorb as much water as possible, even at the expense of a potentially abnormal sodium balance.

But to understand this, we need to talk about water and sodium regulation. If we understand how sodium and water balance is regulated during a normal physiologic state, then we will better understand how dehydration and this change in ADH regulation can lead to hyponatremia.

What are the main functions of aldosterone and ADH?

Aldosterone targets sodium reabsorption, primarily effecting overall fluid status, whereas ADH targets water/fluid reabsorption, primarily effecting sodium levels.

If aldosterone regulates the reabsorption of sodium in the collecting duct of the kidneys, how does this action effect overall fluid status?

Water follows sodium. And because water follows sodium, the sodium level overall will not change. Instead, the overall fluid status changes because of the reabsorption of sodium followed by water.

In contrast, ADH directly regulates water reabsorption in the collecting duct of the kidneys.

How does this action effect overall sodium levels?

If you add free water to a jar filled with salt and water, you will alter the sodium concentration of that jar. The fluid will become more dilute. By this mechanism, shifts in free water absorption mediated by ADH will alter sodium levels. ADH reabsorbs fluid with the goal of altering sodium concentrations, not volume.

While it is true that free water reabsorption should still alter volume to some degree, we are taught that this volume is inconsequential and will ultimately be regulated by aldosterone.

In cases of severe hypovolemia, the goals of ADH shift.

Hyponatremia occurs because of a shift in ADH regulation from sodium to volume. If we think back to the example of the jar filled with salt and water, the fluid will become more dilute with a lower sodium concentration. Volume become the sole focus in an effort to rectify the hypovolemia at the expense of sodium concentrations.

Reviewing the pathophysiology can help us to understand how dehydration can present as both hypo- and hyper-natremia. And while hypernatremia is almost always a result of dehydration, interpreting hyponatremia can be a little more complicated.

Hypovolemic	Euvolemic	Hypervolemic
Diarrhea	SIADH	CHF
Vomiting	Hypothyroidism	Cirrhosis
Pancreatitis	Glucocorticoid deficiency	Nephrotic syndrome
Burns		Acute renal failure
Diuretic induced		Chronic renal failure
Mineralocorticoid deficiency		
Salt-wasting nephropathy		
Cerebral salt wasting		

FIGURE 1-2 **Causes of Hyponatremia.** Examples of etiologies of hypovolemic, euvolemic, and hypervolemic hyponatremia. CHF, congestive heart failure; SIADH, the syndrome of inappropriate secretion of antidiuretic hormone. (Reproduced with permission from Hall JB, Schmidt GA, Kress JP. *Principles of Critical Care*, 4th ed. McGraw Hill, 2015.)

Causes of hyponatremia can be broken up into three categories: Hypovolemic, euvolemic, and hypervolemic hyponatremia (Figure 1-2).

Yet again, understanding the pathophysiology behind each category will put you in the best position to reason through and answer related questions correctly.

Hypovolemic hyponatremia is the most straightforward category. As we discussed, dehydration can present as both hypo- and hypernatremia depending on the severity of the dehydration and behavior of ADH.

Euvolemic hyponatremia is also fairly straightforward. Most commonly, euvolemic hyponatremia is a result of Syndrome of Inappropriate ADH (SIADH) or psychogenic polydipsia.

Psychogenic polydipsia tends to be an easier diagnosis to identify. There will often be a clue related to behavioral problems or tendencies that suggest this diagnosis. While questions certainly come up on the topic, this tends to be lower yield.

SIADH, on the other hand, tends to be higher yield. The most complicated aspect of questions related to euvolemic hyponatremia will more likely be identifying the cause of a patient's SIADH. SIADH can occur as a result of a drug side effect, a sign of malignancy, or secondary to pulmonary pathology (Figure 1-3).

Why do we see euvolemic hyponatremia in SIADH?

Mechanistically, excess ADH will result in excess free water reabsorption. This will dilute overall sodium concentrations.

If we are reabsorbing excess water, why does or doesn't this cause hypervolemia?

Central nervous system diseases	Stroke, hemorrhage, vasculitis, tumor, trauma, infection
Malignancies	Small cell carcinoma of the lung (most commonly associated), cancers of the pancreas and bowel, lymphoma
Inflammatory lung diseases	Infection (eg, pneumonia, lung abscesses, tuberculosis), bronchiectasis, atelectasis, acute respiratory failure, positive-pressure ventilation
Endocrine	Hypothyroidism, adrenal insufficiency
Others	Acute psychosis, pain, postoperative state, severe hypokalemia
Idiopathic	Advanced age can be a risk factor for SIADH

FIGURE 1-3 **Diseases Associated with Syndrome of Inappropriate Antidiuretic Hormone (SIADH).** Central nervous system and lung diseases or malignancies are the most common diseases associated with SIADH. (Reproduced with permission from Walter LC, Chang A, Chen P et al. *Current Diagnosis & Treatment: Geriatrics*, 3rd ed. McGraw Hill, 2021. Data from Fried LF, Palevsky PM. Hyponatremia and hypernatremia, *Med Clin North Am.* 1997 May;81(3): 585–609.)

Aldosterone can still respond appropriately to excrete the excess volume. However, this will do nothing to resolve the abnormal sodium levels. This is why we will remain euvolemic with hyponatremia.

Hypervolemic hyponatremia tends to be the most complicated category.

In what scenarios would you expect to see hypervolemic hyponatremia?

In this case, the problem is with volume regulation. While SIADH is a failure of ADH to regulate sodium levels, hypervolemic hyponatremia results from a failure to adequately regulate volume. The problem lies in "third spacing."

"Third spacing" refers to the fluid extravasation from the intravascular space to a space outside of the circulatory system, known as the interstitial space.

Why does third spacing happen? (Figure 1-4)

Oncotic pressure from osmoles is one of the main forces that maintains fluid volume in the intravascular space. Remember that water follows osmoles. A depletion of osmoles in the intravascular space, particularly albumin, results in a loss of fluid volume to the interstitial space. This is one reason we might see third spacing.

Oncotic forces are opposed by hydrostatic forces. Hydrostatic forces are a result of pressure from the volume in the intravascular space. The higher the hydrostatic pressure, the more likely volume is to leak into the interstitial space. If a patient is volume overloaded, then the higher hydrostatic pressure in the intravascular space results in increased fluid losses to the interstitium.

The capillary membrane also serves to keep fluid within the intravascular space. But in states of increased capillary permeability, fluid is more likely to diffuse across the vascular membrane.

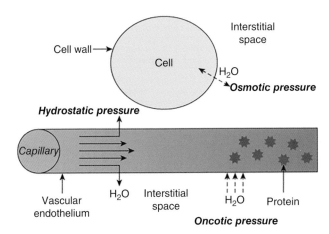

FIGURE 1-4 **Intravascular Hydrostatic and Oncotic Forces**. Protein acts as the major osmole in the vasculature to retain fluid volume. Hydrostatic pressure as a result of the fluid volume opposes the oncotic pressure. The vascular endothelium is a semipermeable membrane that acts as a gatekeeper for fluid and molecules that want to pass between the intravascular and interstitial space. Abnormalities with oncotic or hydrostatic pressure or the vascular endothelium can result in third spacing and edema. (Reproduced with permission from Tenenbein M, Macias CG, Sharieff GQ et al. *Strange and Schafermeyer's Pediatric Emergency Medicine*, 5th ed. McGraw Hill, 2019.)

Why is third spacing problematic?

Fluid in the interstitial space is not part of our "effective circulating volume." The body can only "effectively" use volume within the intravascular space. Because of this, we may see signs and symptoms commonly seen in hypovolemia, such as decreased urine output and/or a rising creatinine. But we can also see signs and symptoms of volume overload due to third spacing, such as pulmonary and pedal edema.

Recall that intravascular volume is an important measure for volume regulation by the kidneys via the glomeruli. If reduced intravascular volumes arrive to the kidneys due to this extravasation to the interstitial space, then the kidneys will operate as though the body is in a hypovolemic state. The same mechanism that occurs in hypovolemic hyponatremia occurs here, except that the body is actually volume overloaded in the "third space."

Can you think of some conditions that lead to edema and third spacing?

The major conditions that you should think of when you see hypervolemic hyponatremia are heart failure, pulmonary edema, and liver failure.

Recall how these conditions are all interconnected. If we think about circulation as a highway, left heart failure will result in reduced ability for the heart to pump blood to the systemic circulation. Any blood backed up in the left heart will eventually back up in the pulmonary system, then the right heart, and eventually to the liver.

Now that we have discussed the various etiologies that can result in hyponatremia, we should discuss specific lab values that might help us to pinpoint one of those etiologies.

What lab values suggest hypovolemia?

Because the kidneys help to regulate volume, kidney function can provide important clues about volume status.

How do kidneys regulate volume status?

In the case of hypovolemia, low intravascular volume in the kidneys triggers the Renin-Angiotensin-Aldosterone System to stimulate increased renal water reabsorption. But in the case of severe hypovolemia, the kidneys will sacrifice themselves for the sake of more vital organs. To do this, the afferent arteriole, which brings blood from the rest of the body to the kidneys, will constrict (Figure 1-5). This allows the redistribution of blood volume to the rest of the body and away from the kidneys.

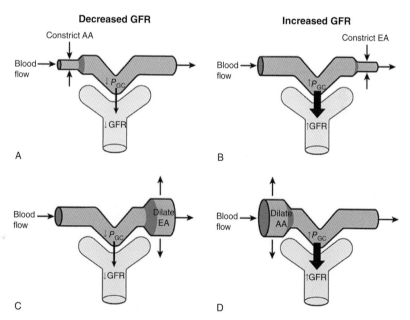

FIGURE 1-5 **Afferent and Efferent Arteriole Effects on GFR.** A: Constriction of the afferent arteriole (AA) results in decreased renal blood flow for filtration at the glomerulus and a decreased GFR. B: Constriction of the efferent arteriole (EA) results in a narrower outflow tract. That pressure results in an increase in renal blood flow filtration through the glomerulus. C: Dilation of the EA results in less pressure force on the renal blood flow to pass through the glomerulus. More renal blood flow passes through the dilated EA. D: A dilated AA results in more renal blood flow delivery to the glomerulus, resulting in an increased GFR. (Reproduced with permission from Widmaier EP, Raff H, Strang KT. *Vander's Human Physiology*, 11th ed. McGraw Hill, 2008.)

How can we use the creatinine and BUN to tell us more information about the etiology of renal disease?

Recall that renal injury can be broken up into three categories: Prerenal, intrinsic renal, and postrenal kidney injury (Figure 1-6).

Prerenal kidney injury is a result of hypovolemia. This is the scenario described above, when the afferent arteriole constricts, reducing blood supply to the kidneys and resulting in kidney injury. Recall that hyponatremic hypervolemia results in a low effective circulating volume, and that prerenal kidney injury may also be seen in the case of "third spacing."

Intrinsic renal injury refers to any pathology and/or injury related to the kidney infrastructure themselves, such as glomerulonephritis or acute tubular necrosis. In intrinsic renal disease, the kidneys cannot function normally due to an intrinsic problem.

Postrenal kidney injury refers to any pathology that physically obstructs urine excretion. This urine backflow will increase pressure on the kidneys and result in renal injury. Obstruction can occur at any point from the ureters to the urethra. Some examples include renal stones, obstructive tumors in the ureter, pelvis, or bladder, or prostate hyperplasia. Obstruction from proximal abdominopelvic structures can also result in postrenal kidney injury. If urine excretion is obstructed, then the excess urine will start to backflow towards the kidneys and cause renal damage.

A BUN/creatinine ratio greater than 20:1 suggests a prerenal etiology (Figure 1-7).

Can you think of a reason why a higher ratio reflects a prerenal etiology?

If severe dehydration is present, then the kidneys will reabsorb as much water as possible. Urea is a major osmole for water reabsorption in the kidneys. If the kidneys are reabsorbing much more water than usual, then a disproportionate amount of urea will also be reabsorbed. This will result in a disproportionately high ratio of BUN to creatinine.

If the ratio is less than 20:1, then an intrinsic or postrenal process is more likely. Other labs and clinical clues will help guide you as to the diagnosis. In the setting of other electrolyte abnormalities, an intrinsic renal pathology is more likely.

Now we have three tools to assess fluid status: Sodium level, creatinine, and the BUN/creatinine ratio. These lab results should be combined with key signs from the vitals and physical exam, such as increased heart rate and dry mucous membranes, to help shape your differential diagnoses.

Remember, interpretation of labs and/or information as a whole, rather than in parts, will strengthen your confidence, accuracy, and test-taking skills. This is especially important in cases of acid-base abnormalities.

After assessing fluid status, I recommend evaluating acid-base status. When abnormal, acid-base status is highly informative and will narrow your differential. Acid-base status can even help to clarify the etiology of an abnormal fluid status.

Prerenal
Decreased intravascular volume
Dehydration
Hemorrhage
Burns
Diuretics
Decreased cardiac output
Heart failure
Arrhythmias
Vascular changes (peripheral vasodilation and/or renal vasoconstriction)
Sepsis
Anaphylaxis
Antihypertensives
Nonsteroidal anti-inflammatories
Intrinsic
Tubular injury/Acute tubular necrosis
Hypotension
Prolonged ischemia
Nephrotoxins
Drugs: aminoglycosides, cyclosporine, amphotericin B, cisplatin
Toxins: ethylene glycol, heavy metals
Pigments: hemolysis, rhabdomyolysis
Interstitial disease
Acute interstitial nephritis
Infection
Malignant infiltrations
Vascular disease
Hemolytic uremic syndrome
Vasculitides (e.g. Wegener granulomatosis)
Thrombosis
Glomerulonephritis
Postinfectious glomerulonephritis
Systemic lupus erythematosus
Membranoproliferative glomerulonephritis
IgA nephropathy
Henoch-Schönlein purpura
Goodpasture syndrome
Postrenal (Obstructive)
Bladder calculi
Posterior urethral valves
Bladder catheter obstruction
Neurogenic bladder

FIGURE 1-6 Differential Diagnoses for Prerenal, Intrinsic Renal, and Postrenal Causes of Acute Renal Failure. Prerenal causes of acute renal failure result in kidney damage because of decreased blood flow to the kidneys. Intrinsic renal disease refers to disease that damages the kidneys directly. Postrenal causes of acute renal failure result in kidney damage due to obstruction downstream from the renal pelvis, resulting in a backflow of urine that can damage the kidneys. (Reproduced with permission from Zaoutis LB, Chiang VW. *Comprehensive Pediatric Hospital Medicine*, 2nd ed. McGraw Hill, 2018.)

Laboratory Test	Prerenal AKI	Intrinsic AKI	Postrenal AKI
Urine sediment	Hyaline casts, may be normal	Granular casts, cellular debris	Cellular debris
Urinary RBC	None	2–4+	Variable
Urinary WBC	None	2–4+	1+
Urine Na (mEq/L or mmol/L)	<20	>40	>40
FE_{Na} (%)	<1	>2	Variable
Urine/serum osmolality	>1.5	<1.3	<1.5
Urine/S_{cr}	>40:1	<20:1	<20:1
BUN/S_{cr} (urea/S_{cr}, SI)	>20 (>100)	~15 (~60)	~15 (~60)
Urine specific gravity	>1.018	<1.012	Variable

FIGURE 1-7 **Comparison of Laboratory Findings for Acute Kidney Injury**. The most important laboratory finding to compare prerenal acute kidney injury (AKI) with intrinsic or postrenal AKI is the BUN/Cr ratio. While the fractional excretion of sodium (FE_{Na}) is also useful, it is uncommonly tested on the USMLE Step 2 exam. AKI, acute kidney injury; BUN, blood urea nitrogen; FE_{Na}, fractional excretion of sodium; S_{cr}, serum creatinine; RBC, red blood cell; WBC, white blood cell.
(Reproduced with permission from DiPiro JT, Yee GC, Posey M et al. *Pharmacotherapy: A Pathophysiologic Approach*, 10th ed. McGraw Hill, 2017.)

If there are signs of dehydration, how would the acid-base status be useful?

A normal acid-base status in the setting of hypovolemia might suggest dehydration from decreased oral intake or minor GI losses, third spacing, poor renal concentrating abilities and/or excessive urination, or hemorrhage.

An abnormal acid-base status in the setting of hypovolemia can suggest a number of etiologies. Hypovolemia itself can sometimes cause a "contraction alkalosis," though this is not commonly tested. Alkalosis can also be seen in cases of excess vomiting due to the loss of hydrogen chloride. In contrast, significant diarrhea and loss of bicarbonate in the stool can result in a nongap acidosis.

What about interpretation of abnormal acid-base status in general?

It is important to have a strategy for interpreting the acid-base status (Figure 1-8). I recommend starting with the bicarbonate. This is the easiest value to interpret. If the bicarbonate is low, then we should be most worried about a metabolic acidosis.

Metabolic acidosis tends to be the highest yield acid-base abnormality. If you are going to memorize only one piece of information about acid-base status, it would be knowing that a metabolic *acidosis* results in low bicarbonate and carbon dioxide levels. Using this as an anchor, you can remember that a respiratory acid-base disturbance is reversed, meaning a low bicarbonate suggests a respiratory *alkalosis*. And if low bicarbonate suggests a metabolic *acidosis*, then a high bicarbonate should suggest a metabolic *alkalosis* and a respiratory *acidosis*.

But test-taking skills should focus on reasoning and avoid memorization.

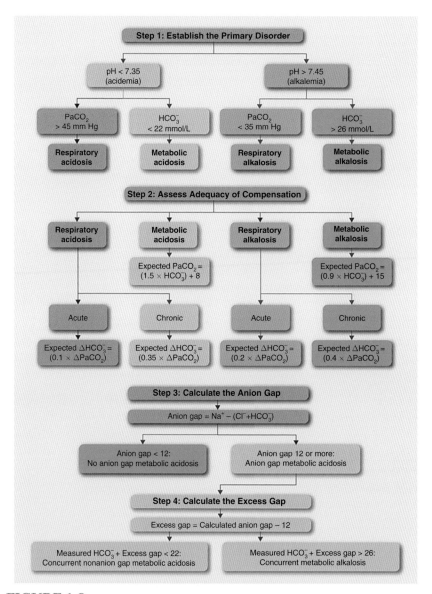

FIGURE 1-8 Approach to Acid-Base Disorders. (Reproduced with permission from Chisholm-Burns MA, Schwinghammer TL, Malone PM et al. *Pharmacotherapy Principles & Practice*, 5th ed. McGraw Hill, 2019.)

Can we reason through why bicarbonate and carbon dioxide would be low in a metabolic acidosis?

If there is excess acid from a metabolic process, then the body will attempt to compensate through two mechanisms: Respiration and renal excretion.

Respiration is the quickest compensatory mechanism. If we want to increase our pH, then we want to blow off an excess of carbon dioxide. This will result in a lower-than-normal level in the blood.

Renal excretion as a compensatory mechanism takes a few days. The biggest clue that renal compensation has occurred is that the pH is only mildly abnormal.

Why is the bicarbonate low in the case of a metabolic acidosis?

Bicarbonate is a buffer in the blood stream and will be used to buffer the excess acid to generate carbon dioxide.

If we are worried about a metabolic acidosis, then we should calculate an anion gap. An elevated anion gap will narrow your differential.

How do you calculate the anion gap?

Subtract bicarbonate and chloride from the sodium level to get your anion gap.

The presence of an anion gap generally suggests the presence of a metabolic, rather than respiratory, acidosis. The most common etiologies for a gap acidosis are lactic acidosis from sepsis and diabetic ketoacidosis. Common things being common, these will always jump to the top of my differential when I see a gap acidosis.

Recall the MUDPILERS mnemonic for causes of gap acidosis: Methanol, urea, diabetic ketoacidosis, propylene glycol, iron or INH, lactic acidosis, ethanol or ethylene glycol, rhabdomyolysis or renal failure, and salicylates (Figure 1-9).

A nongap acidosis usually has a narrower differential. The most common causes of a nongap acidosis include diarrhea or renal tubular acidosis (Figure 1-10).

- Methanol
- Uremia
- Diabetic ketoacidosis
- Paraldehyde
- Iron, isoniazid, inhalants
- Lactic acidosis
- Ethanol, ethylene glycol
- Salicylates

FIGURE 1-9 Differential Diagnosis of Anion Gap Metabolic Acidosis: MUDPILES Mnemonic. (Reproduced with permission from Cydulka R, Fitch MT, Joing SA et al. *Tintinalli's Emergency Medicine Manual*, 8th ed. McGraw Hill, 2018.)

	Type 1 (Distal)	Type 2 (Proximal)	Type 4
Basic defect	Decreased distal acidification	Diminished proximal HCO_3^- reabsorption	Aldosterone deficiency or resistance
Etiology	Autoimmune disease, genetic, medication	Light chain excretion, genetic, medication, idiopathic	Diabetes mellitus, medication, adrenal insufficiency, genetic
Urine pH	>5.3	Variable: >5.3 if above reabsorptive threshold; <5.3 if below	Usually <5.3
Plasma [HCO_3^-], untreated	Often extremely low, 10 mEq/L	Usually 14–20 mEq/L	Usually >15 mEq/L
Fractional excretion of HCO_3^- at normal plasma [HCO_3^-]	<3% in adults; may reach 5–10% in young children	>15–20%	<3%
Plasma [K^+]	Usually reduced, although a hyperkalemic form exists	Usually reduced	Elevated
Dose of HCO_3^- to normalize plasma [HCO_3^-], mEq/kg per day	1–2 in adults; 4–14 in children	10–15	1–3; may require no alkali if hyperkalemia corrected
Nonelectrolyte complications	Nephrocalcinosis, nephrolithiasis, osteopenia	Rickets or osteomalacia	None

FIGURE 1-10 Characteristics of Renal Tubular Acidosis. (Reproduced with permission from Hammer GD, McPhee SJ. *Pathophysiology of Disease: An Introduction to Clinical Medicine*, 8th ed. McGraw Hill, 2019.)

Acid-Base Disorder	Primary pH Change	Pco$_2$ Change	Expected Compensation	Common Causes	Therapy
Acute respiratory acidosis	↓	Pco$_2$ ↑	HCO$_3^-$ ↑1/↑ 10 in Pco$_2$	Narcotics, acute or acute-on-chronic lung disease	Therapy of lung disease, mechanical ventilation, specific antidotes
Chronic respiratory acidosis	↓	Pco$_2$ ↑	HCO$_3^-$ ↑3.5/↑10 in Pco$_2$	Chronic lung disease	Therapy of lung disease
Acute respiratory alkalosis	↑	Pco$_2$ ↓	HCO$_3^-$ ↓2/↓10 in Pco$_2$	Fever, pain, anxiety, mechanical ventilation	Sedation, analgesia, antipyretics
Chronic respiratory alkalosis	↑	Pco$_2$ ↓	HCO$_3^-$ ↓5/↓10 in Pco$_2$	Chronic liver disease, pregnancy, aspirin overdose, and sepsis (with metabolic acidosis)	Therapy of underlying disease

FIGURE 1-11 **Characteristics of Respiratory Acid-Base Disorders**. Respiratory acidosis refers to a state of increased carbon dioxide resulting in decreased pH. Respiratory alkalosis refers to a state of decreased carbon dioxide resulting in increased pH. (Reproduced with permission from Lerma EV, Rosner MH, Perazella MA. *Current Diagnosis & Treatment: Nephrology & Hypertension*, 2nd ed. McGraw Hill, 2018.)

A respiratory acidosis results from excess carbon dioxide intake and should be relatively easy to identify with clinical clues from the vignette. Additionally, we would not expect many other lab values to be abnormal, if any.

Is excess carbon dioxide caused by hyper- or hypoventilation?

I remember the answer to this by using the pH scale as my reference point.

Hyper- refers to excess or high levels, and hypo- refers to less or low levels. In the case of hyperventilation, this increased ventilation results in an increased pH. A higher pH represents an alkalosis. In contrast, decreased ventilation in the case of hypoventilation results in a decreased pH level. A low pH level represents an acidosis. This is a very straightforward way to remember the difference between the two (Figure 1-11).

Compared to acidosis, alkalosis is very uncommon on board exams. The most common causes for alkalosis are from dehydration, acid losses in the setting of vomiting, or hyperventilation.

After interpreting the volume and acid-base status, I review the electrolytes and glucose.

Sodium, chloride, bicarbonate, creatinine, and BUN can all be affected by volume and acid-base status, and we discussed the importance and strategy for interpreting these labs together as a whole.

Pseudohyperkalemia
  Marked thrombocytosis or leukocytosis with release of intracellular K+
  Repeated fist clenching during phlebotomy, tourniquet application, use of small-bore needles during lab draw
Shift of K$^+$ out of the cell
  Metabolic acidosis
  Insulin deficiency
  Hyperglycemia
  α-Adrenergic stimulation
  Tissue injury (rhabdomyolysis, hemolysis, tumor lysis)
  Hyperkalemic periodic paralysis
  Drugs (digoxin overdose, succinylcholine)
Kidney disease, acute and chronic
  Renal secretory defects (may or may not have reduced kidney function): kidney transplant, interstitial nephritis, systemic lupus erythematosus, sickle cell disease, amyloidosis, obstructive nephropathy
Hypoaldosteronism
    Addison disease
    Type IV renal tubular acidosis
    Heparin
    Ketoconazole
  Drugs that inhibit potassium excretion: spironolactone, eplerenone, drospirenone, NSAIDs, ACE inhibitors, angiotensin II receptor blockers, triamterene, amiloride, trimethoprim, pentamidine, cyclosporine, tacrolimus
Excessive intake of K$^+$
  Especially in patients with diminished kidney excretion

FIGURE 1-12 **Causes of Hyperkalemia**. ACE, angiotensin-converting enzyme; NSAIDs, nonsteroidal anti-inflammatory drugs. (Reproduced with permission from Papadakis MA, McPhee SJ, Rabow MW. *Current Medical Diagnosis & Treatment 2021*. McGraw Hill, 2021.)

An abnormal potassium level is rarely explained by an abnormal volume or acid-base status, though there are a few exceptions (Figures 1-12 and 1-13). An abnormal potassium level should increase your suspicion for etiologies such as renal failure, rhabdomyolysis, diarrhea, medication side effect, or ingestion.

And while total body stores of potassium are decreased in diabetic ketoacidosis, the potassium levels on a metabolic panel are often normal.

Why do we lose our total body potassium stores in diabetic ketoacidosis?

Acidosis drives potassium out of the cells and into the intravascular space. The total body stores of potassium become available to be excreted by the kidneys. Excess potassium is lost as the kidneys try to excrete hydrogen ions in the setting of acidosis and osmotic urination.

While there are several other lab tests and values you will encounter, these are by far the highest yield and the most important for your performance on test day.

The goal is to learn how to master the reasoning and pathophysiology needed to excel at lab value interpretation. Practice a methodological approach to interpretation and start to notice patterns as you develop your illness scripts.

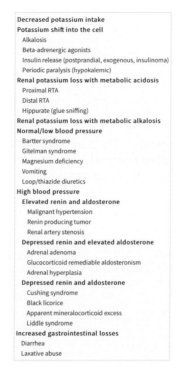

FIGURE 1-13 **Causes of Hypokalemia**. (Reproduced with permission from Papadakis MA, McPhee SJ, Rabow MW. *Current Medical Diagnosis & Treatment 2021*. McGraw Hill, 2021.)

SUMMARY

1. Use a systematic approach.
2. Improve your ability to reason through lab abnormalities by understanding the underlying pathophysiology.
3. Separate concepts into more manageable subcategories.
4. Review and interpret lab findings as a whole, rather than in discreet parts.
5. Incorporate lab value patterns as you develop your illness scripts.

■ SECTION 3: UNDERCONFIDENCE

Underconfidence is an obvious weakness in test-taking. But what can be done?

If you were to enter into combat, having the necessary weapons to defeat your opponent would probably boost your confidence level. Having the necessary tools and test-taking skills for your next board exam should have a similar effect. Already, by reading this book, you are better equipped to conquer the exam.

Part of boosting our confidence also involves altering our expectations about and perception of our performance.

We can't know or remember everything about everything. It is important to come to terms with the fact that you will likely get *many, many* questions wrong in your lifetime. But so will a lot of other people.

All board exams are curved. So, even if you feel like you are only answering 50% of the exam correctly, there is no way to correlate your perceived performance with your actual score. This is important to remember if you start to worry during an exam. That worry will only serve to cloud your judgment for future questions and may be totally unfounded.

Part of our challenge as test-takers is to remain resilient during an exam despite the all-too-common fear that we are failing. We need to maintain confidence that we have done and are doing enough to get the score that we want.

How can we maintain confidence on an exam when we feel we don't know enough?

We are often highly focused on what we *don't* know, when really we should focus on what we *do* know. While we need to collect enough information to support our hypotheses, we don't need to understand or know the significance of every piece of information in the vignette. Only enough to take our best guess.

One weakness for the underconfident is the use of the process of elimination.

Consider the student who uses the process of elimination to arrive at an answer. Even when they think they know the correct answer, they don't feel assured until they can eliminate all the other answer choices.

Elimination is a strategy so many of us are taught in high school and college. But college and medical school are entirely different beasts, and there is no possible way to learn everything for your board exams the way you may have been able to in the past.

The process of elimination relies on some degree of certainty to rule out other answer choices. The less you know overall, the less useful this strategy is. Because of this, the reliability of the process of elimination diminishes on medical board exams, where there is just too much information to know.

In fact, if you arrive at an answer choice that is less familiar to you, the process of elimination may actually influence you to choose that answer because of your inability to rule it out. While you may think that the knowledge you have about the correct answer should protect you, this is not always necessarily true. I have seen students talk themselves out of the correct answer and convince themselves to choose the less familiar choice.

I often tell students that the unfamiliar answer choices are typically not the correct answer. Why?

We tend to know more about the higher yield material. If you have studied enough, then any unfamiliar answer choice is most likely low yield. Correct answers are typically concepts that test writers want you to know well, and those concepts tend to be the high yield concepts. Low yield concepts are low yield for a reason.

For those who struggle with confidence, we want to avoid approaches that will challenge our confidence, like the process of elimination.

Try to avoid comparing yourself to others, worrying about practice scores, or worrying about your score on exam day. These behaviors are tempting but serve no purpose. Remember that test-taking strategies will serve as the best defense.

Let's work through a practice question that might be challenging for those who feel underconfidence is a weakness.

Question

An 8-year-old boy is brought to clinic because of worsening academic perfor-mance. Over the past few months his grades have been declining. He reports that he has been tired lately and his teachers have reported that he sometimes falls asleep during class. He sleeps 9 hours each night and they have not heard any snoring while he sleeps. His parents let him bring his phone to bed at bed-time. He often wakes up with only a few minutes to get ready and get to school. Lately, he has also complained of intermittent constipation. He has no signifi-cant past medical history. His prenatal and delivery course were unremarkable. Vitals are within normal limits. Weight is in the 50th percentile. He appears unengaged with the examiner and remains seated during the encounter. The patient has difficulty opening his hands after squeezing the examiner's fingers. There is full range of motion in the bilateral extremities. Which of the following is the most likely explanation for his presentation?

   a. Attention deficit hyperactivity disorder
   b. Major depressive disorder
   c. Cerebral palsy
   d. Myotonic dystrophy
   e. Poor sleep hygiene
   f. Narcolepsy

Before we start working through this question, do you know why I picked this example for the section on underconfidence?

Initially, this vignette seems rather straightforward. Most of the answer choices are familiar diagnoses. But at the end of this vignette, there is a sentence about how the patient has difficulty opening his hands after squeezing the examiner's fingers. This finding is fairly unusual. Because it is unusual, it is likely highly specific for a single diagnosis. However, if you do not recognize this finding, then your confidence may begin to precipitously decline.

If we start to panic when we see something unfamiliar, we set ourselves up for failure. Panic negatively impacts our confidence. Without confidence, we are at higher risk of misunderstanding clues in the vignette and of choosing an answer for the wrong reasons. We may even choose to ignore unfamiliar information altogether.

In most cases, if you focus on what you *do* know, you should be able to narrow down the answer choices. As you build your reasoning skills, you should be able to reason through unfamiliar information to increase your probability of choosing the correct answer.

With that in mind, let's start working through this question.

In Chapter 2, we will review a methodological approach to answering questions in detail. For now, we can use an abbreviated version of this approach.

Let's start by reading the first sentence. This will give us some context when reading through the rest of the vignette.

An 8-year-old boy is brought to clinic because of worsening academic performance.

How would you describe the context here?

In this case, we have a relatively young pediatric patient with a complaint of worsening academic performance. This may be the primary problem or may be the sequelae of another problem.

Now that we know the context, let's review the question. This will help to guide our focus as we read the rest of vignette.

Which of the following is the most likely explanation for his presentation?

The question tells us that we need to establish a diagnosis. We shouldn't expect to find the diagnosis within the vignette.

Let's review the answer choices before reading the vignette. There are a limited number of possible correct answer choices, and we should keep these in mind as we narrow our differential. The answer choices read:

a. *Attention deficit hyperactivity disorder*
b. *Major depressive disorder*
c. *Cerebral palsy*
d. *Myotonic dystrophy*
e. *Poor sleep hygiene*
f. *Narcolepsy*

With these simple steps, we have established a road map that will prevent aimless reading and wasting precious time.

The remainder of the vignette reads:

> *Over the past few months his grades have been declining. He reports that he has been tired lately and his teachers have reported that he sometimes falls asleep during class. He sleeps 9 hours each night and they have not heard any snoring while he sleeps. His parents let him bring his phone to bed at bedtime. He often wakes up with only a few minutes to get ready and get to school. Lately, he has also complained of intermittent constipation. He has no significant past medical history. His prenatal and delivery course were unremarkable. Vitals are within normal limits. Weight is in the 50th percentile. He appears unengaged with the examiner and remains seated during the encounter. The patient has difficulty opening his hands after squeezing the examiner's fingers. There is full range of motion in the bilateral extremities.*

Because those suffering from underconfidence can often fall victim to traps by the test writer, let's practice categorizing each sentence as useful, not useful, or a trap. This is a strategy we will review in more detail in Chapter 4.

Over the past few months his grades have been declining.

Category: Useful

Why did the test writer include this?

This sentence tells us the timing of his symptoms. While this decline in academic performance has not come about suddenly over the course of days to weeks, it is still a relatively new change. Otherwise, the fact that his grades have been declining provides no new information to us.

In fact, we could argue that this information could be categorized as a trap. By adding an extra sentence focused on the academic performance, the test writer may be attempting to influence the test-taker to focus on a learning disability as the most likely etiology for his worsening performance. However, this would only be a trap if a learning disability was the incorrect etiology.

He reports that he has been tired lately and his teachers have reported that he sometimes falls asleep during class.

Category: Useful

Why did the test writer include this?

We are now given a possible reason for this patient's academic performance decline. Rather than an academic disability, his decline may be secondary to excessive sleepiness.

He sleeps 9 hours each night.

Category: Useful

Why did the test writer include this?

The fact that he sleeps 9 hours every night suggests that this patient does not have a straightforward reason for his excessive sleepiness. While the vignette starts with a focus on academic performance, the primary symptom here may be sleepiness despite sleeping an adequate number of hours every night. Now we should shift our focus to diagnoses that may lead to excessive sleepiness.

His parents let him bring his phone to bed at bedtime.

Category: Trap

Why did the test writer include this?

This information is intended to direct the test-taker towards choosing poor sleep hygiene as the reason for his sleepiness and poor academic performance (Figure 1-14). The question is whether this is a correct or incorrect assumption.

The correct answer should never require you to make assumptions. If the answer was truly sleep hygiene, there should be enough clear data available for you to arrive at this answer over the other choices.

How likely is this patient's excessive daytime sleepiness is attributable to poor sleep hygiene?

In this case, the test writer explicitly states that the patient sleeps for 9 hours each night. Regardless of whether he engages in poor sleep hygiene habits before bed, he is still getting an adequate amount of sleep. Had the test writer said that the patient goes to bed at 10 p.m. and wakes up at 6 a.m., then perhaps we could question whether the patient was actually falling asleep by 10 p.m. or just staying up late on his phone.

They have not heard any snoring while he sleeps.

Category: Useful

1. Regular morning rising time.
2. Avoid daytime napping or limit to <1 hour in the morning or early afternoon.
3. Exercise during the day but not immediately before bedtime.
4. Avoid caffeine, nicotine, and alcohol in the evening.
5. Avoid excessive fluid intake at night to reduce nighttime urination.
6. Avoid large meals before bedtime, but a light snack may promote sleep.
7. Follow a nighttime routine of preparation for bedtime and wear comfortable bedclothes.
8. Ensure a tranquil nighttime environment, minimizing noise and light and keeping room temperature comfortable.
9. Avoid use of electronic devices before bedtime.

FIGURE 1-14 **Sleep Hygiene Recommendations.** Sleep hygiene refers to healthy sleep habits. Sleep hygiene measures are often recommended for individuals with difficulty falling and/or staying asleep and/or insomnia. (Reproduced with permission from Walter LC, Chang A, Chen P et al. *Current Diagnosis & Treatment: Geriatrics*, 3rd ed. McGraw Hill, 2021.)

Heroic snoring
Nocturia
Witnessed breathing pauses during sleep
Excessive daytime sleepiness
Tongue or tonsillar enlargement
Retrognathia
Large neck circumference (>16 in in women, >17 in in men)

FIGURE 1-15 **Common Features Associated with Sleep Apnea**. Consider sleep apnea as a diagnosis when a patient complains of loud snoring, excessive daytime sleepiness, and/or breathing pauses during sleep. Some exam findings that should increase your suspicion for sleep apnea include tongue or tonsillar enlargement, retrognathia, and/or large neck circumference. These abnormal exam findings all can contribute to airway obstruction. (Reproduced with permission from McKean SC, Ross JJ, Dressler DD, Scheurer DB. *Principles and Practice of Hospital Medicine*, 2nd ed. McGraw Hill, 2017.)

Why did the test writer include this?

Daytime sleepiness can commonly be attributed to sleep apnea. But the typical demographic for sleep apnea is an overweight or obese adult male with a large neck circumference (Figure 1-15). Already, by the demographics alone, we should be less suspicious of sleep apnea. The absence of snoring makes this diagnosis even less likely.

He often wakes up with only a few minutes to get ready and get to school.

Category: Not useful

Why did the test writer include this?

This information might allude to the fact that this patient is overly tired and struggles to wake up on time. But we already know that this patient is excessively tired, so the information provided in this sentence is redundant.

Lately, he has also complained of intermittent constipation.

Category: Useful

Why did the test writer include this?

It's not clear why the test writer included this information at this point. However, this additional symptom is highly specific. Because the test writer chose to include this, we should try to determine why as we continue to read the vignette. We may find that this information is not useful or a trap. But for now, we should treat this information as important as we continue to develop our differential.

Had hypothyroidism been included as one of the answer choices, then this would be a reasonable diagnosis to suspect at this point. While the patient is not of the typical demographic, his new excessive tiredness despite adequate sleep as well as constipation are features of hypothyroidism.

We will ultimately need to decide on an answer choice that can explain both his tiredness and constipation. While we could entertain the possibility that his constipation is not relevant to his presenting symptom, this is less likely to be the case on board exams. More commonly, the diagnosis that we choose should explain every symptom presented in the vignette. If the answer choice cannot explain the constipation, then we should have a reasonable explanation for why the test writer chose to include this symptom in the vignette.

It is okay if we ultimately don't know the relevance of the constipation. As I have said, we can't expect to know everything. If you are not sure what diagnoses would explain his constipation, you can hopefully exclude some answers that are very unlikely to.

He has no significant past medical history.

Category: Not useful

Why did the test writer include this?

Though not useful in this case, it is always important to know the past medical history of any patient you are assessing. And while the presence of a particular medical condition could help to explain some of these symptoms, the absence is not very helpful to narrow our differential.

His prenatal and delivery course were unremarkable.

Category: Useful

Why did the test writer include this?

Preterm birth is a risk factor for cerebral palsy. It is highly unlikely to have undiagnosed cerebral palsy at age 8, and this information about his prenatal and delivery course eliminate a possible risk factor for this diagnosis and should decrease our suspicion further.

Vitals are within normal limits. Weight is in the 50th percentile.

Category: Not useful

Why did the test writer include this?

If abnormalities were present, our differential diagnoses might change. But in the absence of abnormalities, we are not provided with much extra information. None of the answer choices can be ruled out in the absence of a vital sign or weight abnormality.

He appears unengaged with the examiner and remains seated during the encounter.

Category: Trap

Why did the test writer include this?

Disengagement with the examiner in this context is likely intended to hint at depression. But besides worsening academic performance, there are no other features that suggest depression. If we were to anchor on this description of the patient, we might be more inclined to choose major depression as our diagnosis despite not much else to support this diagnosis. Anchoring is a test-taking weakness that will be discussed in more detail in Chapter 5.

The patient has difficulty opening his hands after squeezing the examiner's fingers.

Category: Useful

Why did the test writer include this?

This is a highly unusual physical exam finding. Like his constipation, this specific exam finding should help us to narrow our differential. Unlike the constipation, we can feel certain that this finding is relevant to the chief complaint. A finding as specific and unusual as this would never be an incidental finding on a board exam.

What is the significance of this finding?

Often when we don't recognize something, we are quick to ignore it and/or panic. This panic is a disservice and inhibits our ability to reason our way to the correct answer. Let's try to reason through this exam finding. Detailed strategies for reasoning will be discussed in Chapter 3.

We know this patient can squeeze the examiner's fingers without difficulty. The problem here is his difficulty and delay in opening his hands afterwards. He has no difficulty contracting his muscles but does have difficulty relaxing his muscles.

While we still may not recognize the significance of this yet, we have reasoned through the pathophysiology behind this unusual exam finding. In doing so, we have gotten closer to the diagnosis.

We know that we need to arrive at a diagnosis that can explain difficulty relaxing his muscles, constipation, and excessive daytime sleepiness.

Could the constipation be related to his difficulty relaxing his hand muscles?

If this patient is having difficulty relaxing his hand muscles, then it seems plausible that he might have difficulty relaxing the muscles in his colon and rectum. We can conclude that these two features in his clinical presentation are related.

Remember, we want to try to find a diagnosis that explains every symptom and/or finding in the vignette.

There is full range of motion in the bilateral extremities.

Category: Not useful or trap

Why did the test writer include this?

One of the answer choices, myotonic dystrophy, is not highly tested. Given this, many of us may not be too familiar with the features of this diagnosis.

I also just spent time explaining that unfamiliar answer choices are less likely the correct answer. We can use likelihoods to alter our suspicion, but this is not an absolute rule. We still need to consider this as an answer choice.

Myo- refers to muscle, like in myositis or myocarditis or myofascial pain. *Tonic* is often used to describe something stiff, such as a hypertonic muscle. *Dys-* often refers to dysfunction, and *dystrophy* specifically refers to degeneration of an organ or tissue. We can reasonably deduce that myotonic dystrophy is a disorder involving muscular dysfunction and hypertonicity.

Hypertonic muscular dysfunction sounds like the abnormal exam finding in the vignette.

The test writer's mention that there is a full range of motion may deter you from choosing myotonic dystrophy as a diagnosis, especially if you don't have a solid understanding of myotonic dystrophy. But it is possible to have a disease process that effects relaxation of the muscles without effecting range of motion. This is where reasoning and confidence become so important.

Now that we are done reviewing the vignette, let's remind ourselves of the answer choices.

   a. *Attention deficit hyperactivity disorder*
   b. *Major depressive disorder*
   c. *Cerebral palsy*
   d. *Myotonic dystrophy*
   e. *Poor sleep hygiene*
   f. *Narcolepsy*

We know that we need to choose a diagnosis that can explain his muscular abnormalities. This is the most unusual and specific finding in the vignette. And because this finding is so unusual, we may choose to ignore it altogether if we are feeling underconfident.

Based on the muscular abnormalities alone, we would not be wrong to start to anchor on myotonic dystrophy as an answer choice. But before we do, let's work through the rest of the answers.

Most psychiatric diagnoses will not impact muscular function. While depression can sometimes cause psychomotor retardation or agitation, as well as catatonia, these are not very common symptoms. And while he is unengaged with the examiner, possibly suggesting a depressed mood, this is not enough for a diagnosis. It would therefore be reasonable to exclude attention deficit hyperactivity disorder, major depressive disorder, and poor sleep hygiene from our differential. This leaves us with narcolepsy, cerebral palsy, and myotonic dystrophy.

Keep in mind that the test writer could have built up a case for depression, or another psychiatric diagnosis, in this vignette. And regardless of whether a psychiatric diagnosis is present, this alone could not explain his muscular findings and would therefore be the incorrect answer.

If we are not confident in our reasoning abilities, we might be tempted to choose narcolepsy, especially given this is a more familiar answer choice. Narcolepsy is a reasonable consideration given his excessive daytime sleepiness. He also has some unusual muscular findings. While weakness and paralysis can be associated with narcolepsy, difficulty relaxing muscles is not a classic feature of narcolepsy. Also, narcolepsy would not explain the constipation. If narcolepsy was the correct answer, we might expect a few more features in the vignette to support this diagnosis, such as unintended naps during the day.

Let's now consider cerebral palsy. As mentioned earlier, it would be highly unlikely that this patient was undiagnosed with cerebral palsy until now. That, combined with the fact that the test writer included that this patient has no medical conditions and had an uncomplicated delivery and postnatal course.

But cerebral palsy is also a tempting answer if we are not confident. Cerebral palsy is associated with muscular contractures. We could theorize that the contractures in cerebral palsy are like this patient's difficulty relaxing his hand muscles. But cerebral palsy is associated with chronic contractures, rather than a brief episode during a physical exam.

Finally, let's consider myotonic dystrophy. We know that this diagnosis is not high yield, but based on our reasoning, myotonic dystrophy may be the best answer.

Because myotonic dystrophy is a low yield diagnosis, many of us will not know the features of this disease. But earlier, we used our reasoning skills to make some assumptions about this diagnosis; that myotonic dystrophy is a disorder involving muscular dysfunction and hypertonicity.

Our assumptions about myotonic dystrophy can explain his abnormal exam finding(s).

But how can we explain the patient's excessive daytime sleepiness?

Excessive daytime sleepiness is a common feature of myotonic dystrophy (Figure 1-16). However, I wouldn't expect you to know or memorize this fact. Because myotonic dystrophy is a low yield diagnosis, your time and energy are better spent on higher yield topics and developing your test-taking skills to tackle low yield topics.

System	Symptom
Eye	Cataract, retinal degeneration, ocular hypotonia, ptosis, extraocular weakness
Endocrine	Testicular tubular atrophy; diabetes (rarely clinically significant); sometimes abnormalities of growth hormone and other pituitary functions
Brain	Severe involvement in congenital form; mild mental deterioration frequent in adults; hypersomnia; sleep hypoventilation
Peripheral nerves	Variable and rarely clinically significant; minor sensory loss may occur
Skeletal	Cranial hyperostosis, air sinus enlargement; jaw and palate involvement; tallpes (childhood cases); scoliosis (uncommon)
Skin	Premature balding; calcifying epithelioma
Lungs	Aspiration pneumonia from esophageal and diaphragmatic involvement; alveolar hypoventilation

FIGURE 1-16   Other Systems Involved in Myotonic Dystrophy. Myotonic dystrophy is a form of muscular dystrophy that effects the ability for the muscles to relax. Like other forms of muscular dystrophy, there is also progressive degeneration of the muscles. (Reproduced with permission from Valle DL, Antonarakis S, Ballabio A et al. *The Online Metabolic and Molecular Bases of Inherited Disease.* McGraw Hill, 2019.)

Let's proceed as if we did not know that daytime sleepiness is a feature of myotonic dystrophy.

While we were able to reason through some features of the disease based on the name alone, we wouldn't necessarily be able to reason through the pathophysiology behind excessive daytime sleepiness without more knowledge of myotonic dystrophy. While we wouldn't know if this diagnosis explains his sleepiness, we don't have any reason to believe that it doesn't.

If we were to consider narcolepsy as a possible diagnosis in this case, narcolepsy would explain his excessive daytime sleepiness but not his exam findings. The same is true but reversed for myotonic dystrophy. When we are in this situation, we should focus on the more unusual and specific exam finding. Daytime sleepiness is vague and present in many conditions, but difficulty with muscle relaxation is rare.

What is the correct answer?

Myotonic dystrophy

By remaining confident and using reasoning at various steps throughout this vignette, we were able to decide on myotonic dystrophy as the most likely diagnosis. Remember, you know far more than you think you do. The trick is to access that knowledge and learn how to apply it.

Now that we have finished with this question, I would like to highlight the use of process of elimination. While I used this approach to work through this vignette, I generally recommend against relying on the process of elimination, particularly for those who struggle with underconfidence. As mentioned earlier in this section, if we are unable to explain why an answer choice is wrong, then we might feel inclined to select that choice. Instead, we should choose answers based on whichever answer has the most support. Sometimes, we won't be able to explain why an answer is incorrect. And that can sometimes feel anxiety provoking. Our goal should be to limit anxiety provoking behaviors on test day. I recommend use on a question-by-question basis, only to be used if it will elevate your test performance.

SUMMARY

1. Underconfidence impairs your ability to reason through challenging questions.
2. Test-taking skills should equip you with the confidence to tackle anything.
3. Exams are curved. You won't be able to judge your own test performance on exam day.
4. Practice acceptance when you get questions wrong and avoid rumination. This only slows you down.
5. Learn to identify traps that prey on underconfident test takers.
6. Use the process of elimination wisely and sparingly.

■ SECTION 4: REVIEWING ANSWERS

What is the best way to review your answers on an exam before you submit?

Everyone has their own system. Regardless of the system you choose, I advise against reviewing every answer on an exam.

Why is this a bad idea?

Consider you have finished your exam. There are about 10 minutes remaining to review that exam or section, if you're lucky (or have mastered timing as a test-taking skill). You feel rushed because you want to review all the questions. You also read so many vignettes that you can't remember all the scenarios well, so you need to reread many of the questions again before you review the answers you chose.

This approach sets yourself up for failure. When we are rushed, we are more likely to make mistakes.

Have you ever changed an answer at the last minute, only to find out later that your original answer was correct?

We want to avoid these rushed last-minute decisions on an exam. That isn't smart test-taking.

And what about rereading the vignettes?

While rereading the vignette may remind us of all the pertinent details of the scenario, rereading the vignette may also lead us astray. Instead of devoting time to dissecting the vignette like we should have done initially, we are doing a quick read through. And what if that quick read through falsely alters your perception of the scenario?

Presumably, we are more likely to get the answer right the first time after devoting more attention and energy to the question, rather than when we are during a rushed reread.

Conversely, I am sure many of us have reread a vignette while checking our answers and realized our initial understanding of the vignette was incorrect, often because we missed a key piece of information that was essential in choosing the right answer.

So how do we maximize the benefits of rereading vignettes and reviewing our answers, but minimize the potential pitfalls?

I would like to suggest a system that does just that.

Earlier in this chapter, I discussed strategies for time management. I recommended that you prioritize answering the easiest questions first, and save the most difficult questions for last.

My proposed system for reviewing answers is quite similar. I recommend that you establish a system that allows you to review only some of your answers. Particularly those for the more difficult questions.

If you are saving the more difficult questions for the end, then these vignettes will be the most memorable when you finally get to reviewing your answers. Already, this should put you in a more favorable position.

This strategy for reviewing questions also saves time. You eliminate the need to reread every single vignette. This should give you more time to figure out the answers to those more challenging questions.

But what about those easier questions? Should you not review them at all?

I propose that you practice completing these questions during your first read through and don't return to them later.

This doesn't mean you shouldn't check your answer. But you should check your answer before moving on to the next question, not after completing the entire exam. This means that you select an answer, pause, reflect on your level of confidence with this question, and make changes only at that point. This can serve as your "review" of the question. You are both answering the question for the first time *and* reviewing this question during a single time frame. If after this time frame you decide that you feel confident in your answer choice, then I recommend that you do not return to this question. But if you feel unsure, flag the question and plan to review this question after completing the exam, time permitting.

The threshold that you use to flag a question can be individualized. If I am more than 70% sure in my answer, I do not review that question again. But if you are someone that is never 70% sure in your answers, you may need to use a threshold of 50% for this strategy to be effective. This all depends on your own comfort level.

Those questions that you flag will be your guide for reviewing questions. Only those that are flagged should be reviewed.

You should unflag those questions once you decide that you have chosen the best answer based on the information available to you at that time. Oftentimes, we will remain unsure. But we must acknowledge that we won't answer every question correctly and move on. Remember, we want to avoid rumination whenever possible. These exams are a numbers game, and the more questions you get through, the more likely you are to answer more correctly. Once we reach a certain amount of time and energy on a question, we reach a point of diminishing returns, as discussed earlier.

But when should you change your answer choice?

You should always ask yourself, "Is there new evidence that is driving me to change my answer?" Because if there isn't, then you should probably stick with your original answer choice.

You should always have a specific reason or argument as to why you are changing your answer based on new evidence or a new memory. This is how you can avoid second guessing.

As discussed earlier in this text, our initial instinct is powerful. The longer we spend on a question, the more likely we are to talk ourselves out of it. This often does not work in our favor.

Remember that reviewing your answers can be an excellent strategy if you do so smartly. Establishing your strategy for reviewing answers will be most effective if you self-reflect on the instances where reviewing answers helps and harms you.

We just reviewed some strategies for reviewing answers on an exam.

How should we review the answers to practice questions?

One of the most frequently asked questions on this topic is whether to review answers to questions one-by-one, or after completing an entire block of questions.

Those for completing a block of questions and then reviewing often favor the fact that this mimics a testing environment.

On exam day, you will have to complete a block of 40 questions in a 1-hour time period. In doing your practice questions in this block format consistently, you are theoretically training to excel on the exam.

In my experience, this approach tends to be more beneficial in theory than in practice.

Consider a student with poor time management skills on exams. This would be the type of student that could theoretically benefit from mimicking the testing environment and completing blocks of questions, rather than review after each question.

But is this student's problem merely practice? Or is there something more fundamental to their test-taking approach that needs to be addressed?

I would argue the latter. This student likely needs to develop test-taking skills and learn to apply them in order to improve. But during the process of learning test-taking skills, a single question can sometimes take double, triple, or even ten times as long as what would be typical. Focusing on timing practice before investing the time to develop a strategy is like trying to practice speed typing without first learning how to type. Mastering a skill takes time investment early on. But the early time investment saves an enormous amount of time later.

I recommend that students consistently practice untimed questions early on, with the plan to eventually transition to timed questions after mastering test-taking skills. Many students prefer to split their time between practicing questions untimed and timed. This works, too.

An added benefit, if practicing is untimed, is that there is no reason to wait until the end of a block to review the answers. This allows you to review the explanation immediately after working through a vignette. You will be better able to recall the details of the vignette and learn more from each practice question, not to mention waste less time and energy.

To learn most effectively from reviewing practice questions, you could review and dissect questions as thoroughly as we do in this book. But there are also benefits to practicing hundreds of thousands of questions to expose yourself to as much information as possible presented in all the varying scenarios. This is how you learn to recognize what is high yield. It is important to find a balance between quantity and quality. There is value to the way we review questions, and I recommend adopting those approaches that you find most useful and applying them to your review process. Just not necessarily all the time. Find what works for you.

Your review will help guide your own understanding of your weaknesses. By identifying your weaknesses, you will have a better idea of what to focus on. If your weakness is changing the answer at the last minute, then you might want to work on confidence. If your weakness is mixing up information, you might want to work on your reasoning skills.

In terms of strategies for reviewing specific questions, you should understand the details that led, or should have led, you to the right answer.

With each question you answer correctly, or incorrectly, you should be able to explain to another student why that answer is right after your review. If you can't, then you do not have a reliable understanding of the material and your knowledge may not translate on exam day.[1]

Be sure to pay attention to those questions that you answer correctly. Why?

I have worked with students who often arrive at the correct answer but for the wrong reasons.

Remember, there are only so many variations to a concept, but many ways to ask a question. If your focus is narrowed to the question and answer, you will miss other learning opportunities from those questions that would benefit you later.

There is a wealth of information in every question and your job is to uncover it.

SUMMARY

1. Focus on reviewing your answers to only the most difficult questions.
2. Complete an initial read and reread within the same time frame for less challenging questions. Do not go back to review those answers.
3. Only change your answer if there is new or specific evidence driving you to do so.
4. Use your "flag" tool wisely.
5. Consider reviewing questions one-by-one and untimed to allow time to incorporate new test-taking strategies.
6. Recognize and focus on your test-taking weaknesses.
7. Be able to explain the reasoning behind your answer choice.
8. Challenge yourself to explain why each answer is correct or incorrect.

REFERENCE

1. Andrews MA, Kelly WF, DeZee KJ. Why Does This Learner Perform Poorly on Tests? Using Self-Regulated Learning Theory to Diagnose the Problem and Implement Solutions. *Acad Med.* 2018;93(4):612–615.

The 5-Step Approach

2

INTRODUCTION

What is the best way to approach a test question?

There are many ways to tackle questions. I often teach my own approach to students, and that is the approach detailed in this chapter. But this approach may not work for everyone. Whether you choose to adopt my approach, or develop one of your own, what's important is to have a systematic approach to questions that is consistent and works for you.

Why do we need a systematic approach?

Pretend you are moving into a new house and need to go to buy furniture at Ikea. I would bet that most of you would have a plan before arriving. Many of you would probably have a list of items that you need. Some may even grab a map at the entrance and draw out the path you plan to take. Planning and strategizing ahead of time helps to ensure that all necessary items and furnishings are secured. But for those who arrive to Ikea without a plan, the experience would likely be more chaotic and take longer.

When we have a plan, we are often more successful with whatever we are doing. Test-taking is no different.

My 5-Step Approach to answering questions is the plan in this analogy.

The most important element involved in my approach is the process of pausing to synthesize information. If you ultimately decide not to adopt my approach, I encourage you to at least develop an approach that incorporates this element.

What does it mean to synthesize information, and why is this important?

In general, to synthesize means to combine pieces to make a whole. But from the perspective of test-taking, synthesis will involve summarizing the situation based on all its parts and assigning meaning to the information presented to you.

Let's imagine the following scenario.

A patient comes into your office complaining of fatigue, low energy, difficulty sleeping, and overall achiness. She has no appetite. You might start worrying about cancer, infection, or even an autoimmune disease. As you review her chart, you notice she has a history of major depressive disorder. If you do not pause here and reassess the scenario, you may gloss past this important piece of history.

As we obtain new information, our differential changes. As our differential changes, the information that is most important, and the information that we should pay the most attention to, will change. This is why it is important to periodically pause and synthesize all the information we have before us. With each pause, our perspective may change.

To synthesize information well, we need to learn to assign significance to that information as it relates to the clinical scenario. If this woman had presented with an ankle fracture, then her history of major depression would not be very useful, and we would assign very little importance to it. But in this case, if we were to pause and synthesize the information before us, we would recognize that her symptoms are consistent with major depression.

By pausing to synthesize information and assign importance based on this synthesis, we can better decide what is truly important.

The other element that is essential to consider in synthesizing, or assigning importance to, information is the question in the vignette. The question is the key to determining what is important. It is the foundation of the house you are building. Just as new information will alter the focus of your attention, so will the question.

The fact that I love dogs may be very important to someone who is trying to buy me a gift, but largely uninformative to someone interviewing me for a job.

This is why I encourage students to read the question ahead of time.

So, even if you do not use my approach, my message is this one: Pause to synthesize information while reading the vignette and read the question ahead of time.

Now I will describe my 5-Step Approach.

THE 5-STEP APPROACH

Step 1: Read the last two sentences, then the first two. This includes the question.

The second-to-last sentence typically has the juiciest information, strategically placed there so your tired eyes may miss it by the end of the vignette.

Also, have you ever found yourself reading a vignette, thinking "I know this diagnosis!" only to find it is already stated in the second to last sentence? Your deductive efforts, and time, were wasted.

And as we have discussed, reading the question early on will alter how you attend to the rest of the information in the vignette.

The first and second sentences usually include the context of the scenario.

What do I mean by context?

Context sets the stage. It represents the circumstances of the encounter. Context typically involves the age, gender, health status, chief complaint, and timing.

In my experience, students often neglect the context in these first few sentences. Students quickly read over them, as if the information is unimportant compared to the details of the scenario. But when building a differential, context becomes essential. You cannot begin to assign importance to information without first understanding the context.

Let's review some examples of how and when context is especially relevant in particular conditions or disease states.

Male versus female sex will alter the risk profile:

- Female: Rheumatologic conditions
- Male: Cardiovascular disease or spondyloarthropathies

Ethnicity is often used by test writers to provide context:

- African American: Sickle cell disease, sarcoidosis
- Latinx: Rheumatic fever, tuberculosis, Chagas disease
- Asian: Kawasaki

Age:

- Older: Cancer, vascular disease, chronic conditions
- Younger: Congenital diseases, diseases stemming from infections, osteo-sarcoma, leukemia

Acute or chronic:

- Variable depending on the condition
- Cough example: Acute might suggest pneumonia, whereas chronic might suggest tuberculosis, COPD, or asthma
- Leg pain example: Acute might suggest trauma, whereas chronic might suggest malignancy or arthritis

Now, back to the 5-Step Approach.

Step 2: Interpret and synthesize the information in the vignette to inform a differential.

As mentioned earlier, synthesis will involve summarizing the situation based on all its parts and assigning meaning to the information presented to you.

Think of this step as the opening sentence of your Assessment & Plan.

Step 3: Anchor yourself to an answer before reading the answer choices.

If you don't know the answer, at least try to develop a preliminary conclusion about what you think is going on and/or to generate a road map for the information you think you need to arrive at an answer.

By anchoring before reading the answer choices and the rest of the vignette, you are forced to generate a conclusion based on the four most important sentences. This means you are less likely to be influenced by tempting answer choices and traps in the vignette laid by the test writer. This strategy is especially useful for those plagued by underconfidence.

Step 4: Read the answer choices and try to choose an answer before reading the rest of the vignette, if possible.

Try to choose an answer even if you don't know for sure.

Just like in Step 3, anchoring on an answer choice before you read the remainder of the vignette will reduce the likelihood that you are misguided when you read the remainder of the vignette.

You may find that the answer you generated in Step 3 is not one of those listed. If that happens, you should assess why this is the case. Is it because the test writer was looking for a different type of answer? Did you misunderstand the question?

And even if you are not able to pick an answer yet, this step should still guide how you read the rest of the vignette. As you read the vignette, the conclusion you come up with must match up with one of those answer choices.

If you were not able to pick out an answer at this step, stop reading the vignette when you think you know the answer.

Step 5: Read the rest of the vignette.

Now that you have completed Steps 1–4, you should have the following mindset while reading the rest of the vignette: What information disputes your choice, and what information supports it?

Remember, if you were not able to choose an answer in Step 4, stop reading when you think you know the answer. Then continue reading. Only change your answer if you have new information that goes against your answer choice.

Why am I recommending you stop once you know the answer?

For the same reason as that in Steps 3 and 4; by making a choice and standing by that choice, you are less likely to be influenced by test writer traps and underconfidence as you continue reading.

This completes the 5-Step approach.

Let's apply this approach to some practice questions. Even if you know the answers to these questions, it will still be beneficial to work through the approach in these examples.

Question 1

A 50-year-old African American, nulliparous woman comes to the office for her annual well-woman exam. She feels well overall though she continues to experience hot flashes. She is excited to tell you that she recently lost 10 pounds, which is good news for her upcoming family vacation. She mentions that her menses returned a few months ago, but she was not concerned because the bleeding is irregular and much lighter than before. Prior to this, she had not menstruated in approximately 12 months. She has no chronic medical conditions and takes no medications. Her last Pap smear with human papillomavirus co-testing was normal 3 years ago. BMI is 35 kg/m^2, blood pressure is 120/80 mmHg and pulse is 85/min. Which of the following is the best next step?

a. Pap smear
b. Endometrial biopsy
c. CT Abdomen & Pelvis
d. Prescribe hormone replacement therapy
e. Prescribe sertraline
f. Return next year for annual exam

Step 1: Read the last two sentences, then the first two. This includes the question.

This reads:

BMI is 35 kg/m^2, blood pressure is 120/80 mmHg, and pulse is 85/min. Which of the following is the best next step in management of this patient?

A 50-year-old African American, nulliparous woman comes to the office for her annual well-woman exam. She feels well overall though she continues to experience hot flashes.

What I've learned:

- Middle-aged, African American female
- Nulliparous
- Perimenopausal or menopausal symptoms
- Obese
- Normal vitals
- Well-woman exam

Step 2: Interpret and synthesize the information in the vignette to inform a differential.

Remember, think of this as the opening sentence of your Assessment & Plan.

Interpretation:

- Middle-aged, African American female: Increased likelihood of certain diseases
- Nulliparous: More estrogen exposure
- Perimenopausal or menopausal: Uterine bleeding would be abnormal if menopausal; unlikely bleeding is pregnancy related
- Obese: Increased estrogen exposure; higher risk for metabolic syndrome
- Normal vitals: Reduces likelihood of more acute or infectious diseases
- Well-woman exam: Feeling well overall; not especially bothered by symptoms

What is our synthesis?

50-year-old African American, nulliparous, obese, perimenopausal versus menopausal, asymptomatic female presents for well-woman exam.

Step 3: Anchor yourself to an answer before reading the answer choices.

As a reminder, the question reads:

Which of the following is the best next step in management of this patient?

Based on the four sentences we have read, we do not have enough information to answer this question. We need to read more from the vignette.

Step 4: Read the answer choices and try to choose an answer before reading the rest of the vignette, if possible.

As a reminder, the answer choices read:

a. *Pap smear*
b. *Endometrial biopsy*
c. *CT Abdomen & Pelvis*
d. *Prescribe hormone replacement therapy*
e. *Prescribe sertraline*
f. *Return next year for annual exam*

Though we are not yet sure what is going on with the patient, let's review what we know about the answer choices. This will help to inform the kinds of details that we should pay the most attention to when we go on to read the vignette.

a. *Pap smear*: Pap smear should be done as a cervical cancer screening tool every 5 years until age 65 if normal, and more frequently if abnormal. When we read the vignette, we can pay attention to her history of screening.
b. *Endometrial biopsy*: A major indication for endometrial biopsy is when there is abnormal uterine bleeding. Causes for abnormal uterine bleeding can be remembered with the PALM-COEIN mnemonic, as shown in Figure 2-1. We should look for anything that suggests the patient is experiencing abnormal uterine bleeding. If this patient is menopausal, then any vaginal bleeding would be abnormal.

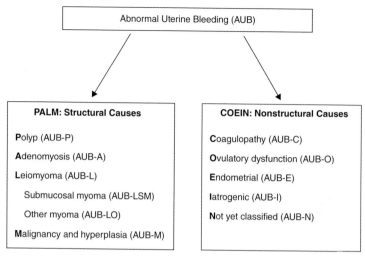

FIGURE 2-1 **PALM-COEIN Classification System.** This system is useful to
remember the causes of abnormal uterine bleeding in nonpregnant women. (Reproduced
with permission from Szymanski LM, Bienstock JL. *The Johns Hopkins Handbook of
Obstetrics and Gynecology*. McGraw Hill, 2016. Data from ACOG. Diagnosis
of abnormal uterine bleeding in reproductive-aged women. Practice Bulletin No. 128,
July 2012.)

   c. *CT Abdomen & Pelvis*: A CT would be useful to evaluate for a mass, though
      ultrasound is usually first line, given its lack of radiation and good visual-
      ization of gynecologic structures. When an answer choice offers a diagnos-
      tic step that is typically not first line, then it is most likely wrong regardless
      of the diagnosis. Because of this, we can lower our suspicion for this answer
      choice.

   d. *Prescribe hormone replacement therapy*: From Step 1, we know that she
      is having hot flashes, but these are not the reason that she has come to
      clinic. She is here for an annual exam. This is an example of when context is
      important. If she was here for help managing her hot flashes, then I would
      be more likely to consider hormone replacement therapy as an answer
      choice, and we may still learn that these symptoms are bothersome enough
      to consider therapy. However, the presence of answer choices that involve a
      diagnostic work-up should raise your suspicion that there will be a different
      focus to this vignette.

   e. *Prescribe sertraline*: Like hormone replacement therapy, sertraline can be
      used for management of menopausal symptoms in addition to depression
      and anxiety. This could be a consideration if we were to consider peri-
      menopausal or menopausal symptom management, as discussed above.
      Additionally, we should pay attention to any mental health symptoms, as
      this would be another indication to prescribe sertraline. However, if this
      patient was indeed depressed, we might expect at least one other answer
      choice as a possible treatment for depression or a psychiatric illness.

Otherwise, this question would not present much difficulty once we had made the diagnosis of major depression.

f. *Return next year for annual exam*: This would require that there were no symptoms requiring diagnostic evaluation or treatment.

Notice how useful reviewing the answer choices can be, even when we do not yet know enough to answer the question. In this case, we were able to use the answer choices, combined with Steps 1–3, to generate a road map that will allow us to read the vignette in a very intentional and directed fashion.

Step 5: Read the rest of the vignette.

Remember, if you were not able to choose an answer in Step 4, stop reading when you think you know the answer. Then continue reading.

The remainder of the vignette reads:

She is excited to tell you that she recently lost 10 pounds, which is good news for her upcoming family vacation. She mentions that her menses returned a few months ago, but she was not concerned because the bleeding is irregular and much lighter than before. Prior to this, she had not menstruated in approximately 12 months. She has no chronic medical conditions and takes no medications. Her last Pap smear with human papillomavirus co-testing was normal 3 years ago.

Because we generated a road map, we should be able to pick out key features from the vignette and assign meaning to those features as they relate to the context and question. Some of the key features in the rest of this vignette are as follows:

Key features:

- Recent weight loss
- Return of menstrual bleeding
- Menopausal (no menses for 12 months)
- Last Pap smear with HPV testing was normal 3 years ago

Significance of key features:

- Recent weight loss: unintentional weight loss should increase suspicion for malignancy or depression
- Return of menstrual bleeding: abnormal uterine bleeding
- Menopausal (no menses for 12 months): abnormal uterine bleeding in menopausal woman is highly concerning for uterine malignancy
- Last Pap smear with HPV testing was normal 3 years ago: given her Pap smear was normal 3 years ago, her abnormal uterine bleeding is less likely related to cervical malignancy. Additionally, she would not be due for another Pap smear for another 2 years.

Now, let's interpret the information we have gathered in a systematic fashion.

There is nothing in the vignette to suggest depression or anxiety. This means that sertraline would only be useful to treat her menopausal symptoms. But

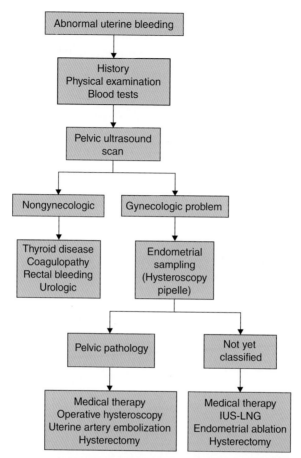

FIGURE 2-2 **Management of Abnormal Uterine Bleeding.** Evaluation for abnormal uterine bleeding should be done in a stepwise manner according to the history gathered. Based on history and blood tests, a pelvic ultrasound may be indicated. Depending on any abnormalities seen, endometrial biopsy is a good next step to evaluate further, particularly in the case of ruling out uterine malignancy. (Reproduced with permission from DeCherney AH, Nathan L, Laufer N, Roman AS. *CURRENT Diagnosis & Treatment: Obstetrics & Gynecology,* 12th ed. McGraw Hill, 2019.)

besides the second sentence, there is no other mention of her menopausal symptoms. This makes it unlikely that menopausal symptom management is the next best step. Given this, we can exclude both sertraline and hormone replacement therapy as possible answer choices.

Her unintentional weight loss is concerning for malignancy. In earlier steps, we identified how her nulliparity and obesity put her at increased risk for estrogen-influenced malignancies such as uterine, ovarian, or breast. The combination of post menopausal uterine bleeding and increased lifetime estrogen exposure should increase your suspicion for uterine cancer. And if we think back to the context of this scenario, her older age is consistent with this diagnosis.

What is the next best step when you are suspicious for uterine malignancy?

If you don't know the answer, you can try to reason through the remaining options. The only answer choices that could diagnose a uterine malignancy are CT or endometrial biopsy.

The best way to evaluate for uterine malignancy is with an endometrial biopsy (Figure 2-2). An endometrial biopsy can be done in clinic, which makes this a reasonable first step in the diagnostic work-up of this patient. An ultrasound can also help to make the diagnosis, but is not an answer choice.

CT may be indicated later for staging but is not the best next step. In fact, a negative CT may not rule out a uterine malignancy, and so we would still need a biopsy for a more definitive answer. This is in contrast to other malignancies, where we typically start the diagnostic work-up with imaging and use biopsies to help make or confirm the diagnosis.

What is the correct answer?

Endometrial biopsy

When developing your illness scripts, you should try to commit to memory the best diagnostic tool for a given condition. Illness scripts will be discussed further in Chapter 4.

Question 2

A 42-year-old woman comes to the office for her annual physical. The patient is feeling well overall except for fatigue that she has experienced most days for several months. She previously visited her grandson every Sunday but has felt too tired to keep up with her usual visits. She lost her job a few months ago, which she also attributes to being less interested in her job and "too tired to focus." The patient tells you that her recent unemployment has caused her to worry about finances. "All this worrying has caused me to lose my appetite! The good news is I've lost 10 pounds without even trying." The patient had previously been trying to lose weight on a vegan diet after being told she was pre-diabetic earlier this year, although her efforts had been unsuccessful until now. Last menstrual period was 2 weeks ago. Her menses have occurred at regular intervals and have always been heavy. Past medical history is also notable for breast cancer, and the patient tells you she has been having trouble sleeping since her cancer diagnosis. Medications include metformin and an aromatase inhibitor. Today, her blood pressure is 110/75 mmHg and heart rate is 85/min. Physical exam is unremarkable. Laboratory and imaging studies done before coming in are unchanged from prior. The patient scores a 23 on the mini-mental status exam done today, compared to a score of 27 done one year ago. What is the most likely cause of her symptoms?

a. Anemia
b. Dementia
c. Vitamin deficiency
d. Cancer recurrence
e. Major depressive disorder
f. Medication side effect
g. Adjustment disorder

Step 1: Read the last two sentences, then the first two. This includes the question.

This reads:

The patient scores a 23 on the mini-mental status exam done today, compared to a score of 27 done one year ago. What is the most likely cause of her symptoms?

A 42-year-old woman comes to the office for her annual physical. The patient is feeling well overall except for fatigue that she has experienced most days for several months.

What I've learned:

- Abnormal mini-mental status exam (MMSE) score
- Normal MMSE score one year earlier
- 42-year-old woman
- Feels well except for fatigue

Step 2: Interpret and synthesize the information in the vignette to inform a differential.

Interpretation:

- Abnormal MMSE score: Clinically significant decline in cognitive function
- Normal MMSE score one year earlier: Relatively new symptoms
- 42-year-old woman: Young for dementia-related memory loss
- Feels well except for fatigue: Narrows your differential

What's our synthesis?

42-year-old woman presents for annual physical with fatigue and memory loss, which are new compared to last year.

Step 3: Anchor yourself to an answer before reading the answer choices.

As a reminder, the question reads:

What is the most likely cause of her symptoms?

The question wants us to focus on her symptoms.

What are her symptoms?

Memory loss and fatigue.

We need to think of possible causes or diagnoses that could result in both fatigue and memory loss.

First, let's build a differential for memory loss:

- Dementia
- Traumatic brain injury
- Medications
- Toxic exposures
- Stroke
- Major depressive disorder
- Vitamin deficiency

Next, let's build a differential for fatigue:

- Anemia
- Malignancy
- Hypothyroidism
- Major depressive disorder
- Medications
- Autoimmune conditions
- Vitamin deficiency

Though these lists are not exhaustive, the only common causes or diagnoses from both lists include medications, vitamin deficiency, and major depressive disorder.

Based on these lists, we can already start to anchor before even reading the answer choices or the rest of the vignette. Just remember to keep an open mind as we get new information. We may need to change our differential if new information alters our degree of suspicion for or against a diagnosis.

Step 4: Read the answer choices and try to choose an answer before reading the rest of the vignette, if possible.

As a reminder, the answer choices read:

a. *Anemia*
b. *Dementia*
c. *Vitamin deficiency*
d. *Cancer recurrence*
e. *Major depressive disorder*
f. *Medication side effect*
g. *Adjustment disorder*

In Step 3, we determined that major depression, a vitamin deficiency, or a medication side effect were the most likely diagnoses based on the information we had available to us. We should feel reassured to see them on the list of answer choices.

When we read the vignette, we should pay special attention to signs of major depression, medications that this patient is taking, and any reasons why she might have a vitamin deficiency.

Without this exercise, if only subtle symptoms were present, we could have missed the diagnosis.

Let's review the answer choices again in detail and try to generate a road map to ready us to read the vignette. As we consider potential causes or associations with each answer choice, we can determine what aspects of the vignette warrant extra attention.

a. *Anemia*
   Think about causes of anemia:
      Diet
      Malignancy
      Rheumatologic disease
      Menorrhagia
      Hemoglobinopathies
      Medications
   Think about signs of anemia:
      Fatigue
      Dizziness
      High-flow systolic cardiac murmur
      Pallor

b. *Dementia*
   Think about causes of dementia:
      Hereditary causes
      Vascular
      Aging
      Spontaneous
      Parkinson's
      Medications
      Alcohol abuse
   Think about signs of dementia:
      Forgetfulness
      Getting lost in familiar places
      Word finding difficulties
      Stepwise progression
      Other vascular diseases

        Visual hallucinations

        Movement disorders

        Heavy alcohol use history

  c. *Vitamin deficiency*

    Think about causes of vitamin deficiency:

        Alcohol abuse

        Extreme diet

        Intestinal abnormalities

        Autoimmune conditions

    Think about signs of vitamin deficiency:

        Poor wound healing

        Dizziness

        Poor vision

        Anemia

        Neuropathy

  d. *Cancer recurrence*

    Think about signs of cancer recurrence:

        Weight loss

        Early satiety

        Signs of metastasis

        New palpable masses

        New blood clot

        Fatigue

        Neurologic symptoms unlikely except in the case of brain metastasis

  e. *Major depressive disorder*

    Think about risk factors for depression:

        History of depression

        Family history of depression

        Aging

        Life stressors

    Think about signs of depression (SIG E CAPS):

        Sleep disturbance

        Interest reduced

        Guilt

        Energy changes

        Concentration decreased

        Appetite changes

        Psychomotor agitation or retardation

        Suicidality

  f. *Adjustment disorder*

    Think about risk factors for adjustment disorder:

        Life stressor(s)

Think about signs of adjustment disorder:

Temporal association of symptoms with life event

Symptoms do not meet criteria for another disorder

g. *Medication side effect*

Medication side effect is a broad category. When we think of a medication side effect, we want to attend to any clues about when the medication was started in relation to symptom onset. Oftentimes, the test writer will be sure to include this temporal association to help guide your answer choice. When you notice this temporal association in a vignette, it is important for you to think about whether this makes "medication side effect" more or less likely, because they are giving you that information to help either rule in or rule out that answer choice.

Step 5: Read the rest of the vignette.

If you were not able to choose an answer in Step 4, stop reading when you think you know the answer. Then continue reading.

The remainder of the vignette reads:

She previously visited her grandson every Sunday, but has felt too tired to keep up with her usual visits. She lost her job a few months ago, which she also attributes to being less interested in her job and "too tired to focus." The patient tells you that her recent unemployment has caused her to worry about finances. "All this worrying has caused me to lose my appetite! The good news is I've lost 10 pounds without even trying." The patient had previously been trying to lose weight on a vegan diet after being told she was prediabetic earlier this year, although her efforts had been unsuccessful until now. Last menstrual period was 2 weeks ago. Her menses have occurred at regular intervals and have always been heavy. Past medical history is also notable for breast cancer, and the patient tells you she has been having trouble sleeping since her cancer diagnosis. Medications include metformin and an aromatase inhibitor. Today, her blood pressure is 110/75 mmHg and heart rate is 85/min. Physical exam is unremarkable. Laboratory and imaging studies done before coming in are unchanged from prior.

For this vignette, let's stop after a few sentences and go through the exercise of synthesizing what we've read and assign meaning as it pertains to our differential diagnosis.

She lost her job a few months ago, which she also attributes to being less interested in her job and "too tired to focus."

Synthesis: Loss of interest and concentration reportedly led to loss of her job. This means that the concentration preceded the job loss. This suggests that an adjustment disorder secondary to the loss of her job is less likely, though still a possibility. Decreased interest and concentration are both criteria for major depression and further support this answer choice.

Differential(s): Major depression or, less likely, adjustment disorder.

The patient tells you that her recent unemployment has caused her to worry about finances.

Synthesis: This sentence is not very useful. The focus is still behavioral. Because we read the answer choices beforehand, we know that the only psychiatric disorders we should be considering are major depression and an adjustment disorder. Excessive worry as seen in generalized anxiety disorder is not an option. Because this information does not add to our differential, we should devote less energy to it.

All this worrying has caused me to lose my appetite!

Synthesis: Loss of appetite.

Differential(s): Loss of appetite can be a sign of some malignancies or major depression as part of the SIG E CAPS criteria. Loss of appetite could also raise your suspicion for a vitamin deficiency, though this would result from the loss of appetite.

The good news is I've lost 10 pounds without even trying.

Synthesis: Unintentional weight loss.

Differential(s): Like loss of appetite, unintentional weight loss should make us think about malignancy, major depression, or a vitamin deficiency.

The patient had previously been trying to lose weight on a vegan diet after being told she was prediabetic earlier this year, although her efforts had been unsuccessful until now.

Synthesis: Weight loss has occurred within the last year. This is a similar timeline to her decreased MMSE score. She tried a vegan diet during the last year, too.

Differential(s): A vegan diet might increase concern for anemia secondary to B12 or iron deficiency. However, the vignette states she was unable to lose weight on a vegan diet, suggesting that this alone cannot explain her unintentional weight loss. Note that anemia *and* vitamin deficiency are possible answer choices, so only one can be the correct answer choice.

Last menstrual period was 2 weeks ago.

Synthesis: Menstrual female with source of regular blood loss. Unlikely to be pregnant.

Differential(s): The relevance here is that she is still menstruating, so anemia from menorrhagia is a possibility.

Her menses have occurred at regular intervals and have always been heavy.

Synthesis: Heavy bleeding, with a source of regular blood loss.

Differential(s): This would provoke concern for anemia, as above.

Past medical history is also notable for breast cancer, and the patient tells you she has been having trouble sleeping since her cancer diagnosis.

Synthesis: History of breast cancer with trouble sleeping since her diagnosis.

Differential(s): Her history of breast cancer suggests that cancer recurrence is a possibility. Because cancer recurrence was listed as an answer choice, we could have already assumed she had cancer in the past and this sentence only confirms our suspicion.

Her difficulty sleeping fulfills another criterion for major depression. The fact that this symptom began after a life stressor might also increase concern for an adjustment disorder.

Medications include metformin and an aromatase inhibitor.

Synthesis: These medications are not very informative because we already have been told about her prediabetes and breast cancer. However, we know that medication side effect is one of our leading differential diagnoses, and we need to consider this as a possible cause of her symptoms.

Could metformin or aromatase inhibitors explain her fatigue and memory loss?

Test writers must give you enough clues to choose the best answer. If there is support for a different answer choice, then this is likely the correct answer.

It would be perfectly fine to guess medication side effect if you could not find evidence to support any other answer choice. But you should be sure that you understood the question correctly before using this approach.

Today, her blood pressure is 110/75 mmHg and heart rate is 85/min. Physical exam is unremarkable.

Synthesis: Normal vitals and physical exam. This doesn't alter our differential.

Physical exam is unremarkable.

Synthesis: The absence of findings does not hold much significance. However, the presence of findings could have been informative, including objective signs of neuropathy or dementia.

Laboratory and imaging studies done before coming in are unchanged from prior.

Synthesis: Just as stated, there have been no changes to her biomarkers.

Differential(s): This should decrease suspicion for anemia or vitamin deficiency, as you would expect to see some abnormalities on routine blood work. And unchanged imaging would suggest that a cancer recurrence is very unlikely.

Now that we've finished reading the remainder of the vignette, let's think back to the answer choices that we were considering. In Step 3, we anchored on a medication side effect, vitamin deficiency, or major depression as possible answer choices.

Hopefully you were able to stop at some point while reading the vignette to anchor on an answer choice. But let's go through how we would arrive at an answer choice after completing Step 5.

We should start by considering whether any diagnoses are well supported by *all* or *most* of her complaints.

This is a very important point. Though it may seem obvious, this is a very common pitfall in practice. When struggling to choose between two diagnoses, your focus should be on which answer can be supported by all or almost all the information presented.

For example, we can consider our differential of major depression versus adjustment disorder, if you were to choose to consider the latter.

If we first consider major depression, we can think through the SIG E CAPS criteria. This patient exhibits features of major depression, including sleep disturbance, lack of concentration, appetite changes, and psychomotor depression. She also describes lack of interest, or anhedonia. Recall that anhedonia or depressed mood are required to make a diagnosis of major depression in adults. Instead of depressed mood, children and adolescents can present with irritability.

If we are considering major depression as our leading differential, we need to make sure that this patient's major symptoms can be explained by this diagnosis.

In this case, can the presence of major depression explain both fatigue and memory loss?

Depression can indeed explain both fatigue and memory loss, though memory loss is more commonly seen in older patients. You may recall that an MMSE score is not considered representative if a patient meets criteria for major depression, as depression can indeed lead to memory loss. This is called pseudodementia.

While you could argue that adjustment disorder could explain her fatigue, this diagnosis could not explain her memory loss.

Because we determined a list of differential diagnoses in earlier steps that did not include adjustment disorder, this diagnosis should be very low on our differential. This should only change if new information was presented that greatly changes our suspicions.

This is where the steps become very helpful. The stepwise approach in this case should protect you from falling into traps set by the test writer. Because while adjustment disorder requires a triggering event, a triggering event does not always lead to an adjustment disorder.

When we are faced with considering a low-yield answer choice like adjustment disorder, the problem is that we tend to know or remember less about those low-yield diagnoses. This means that any low-yield answer choice is an easier trap to fall into, because we may talk ourselves into choosing it due to this gap in knowledge.

In considering the remainder of the answer choices, I propose that you do not need to know why every answer is wrong. You only need to have enough support to select the best answer. If you can explain all or most of the features highlighted in the vignette with an answer choice, then this is probably correct.

Test writers will give you answer choices that are difficult to rule out. For example, a medication side effect is hard to rule out. Who knows *every* side effect of every medication?

Though some of you may be tempted to choose medication side effect as an answer choice if unsure, I would encourage you to remain confident in what you *do* know, rather than what you don't.

If you have enough evidence to support major depression alone as a diagnosis then depression is a more likely choice, even if you do not feel confident enough to rule out other answer choices. While it is always prudent to consider whether the symptoms could be explained by a medical condition or medication when making a psychiatric diagnosis, we need to consider the knowledge we have available to us in the moment and choose the best answer to us at the time.

Whenever we do consider the possibility of a medication side effect, we should determine whether there is a temporal association between the symptoms and the start of the medication. This is an easy strategy to utilize as a test taker and an easy trap to set for the test writer. If there is not a temporal association, then it is highly unlikely that a medication is causing symptoms.

However, there are exceptions to this rule. For example, ACE inhibitors can lead to cough as a side effect at any point in taking the medication. But remember that this is among the exceptions.

In this case, we know that her symptoms started at some point after her cancer diagnosis. Presumably, she also started the aromatase inhibitor shortly after the diagnosis was made. A temporal relationship means that we cannot rule out the possibility. But this does not mean causation.

Another strategy we can use is to try to consider the goals of the test writer with this question.

What is special about this scenario, if anything?

In this case, we have mood complaints and fatigue in the setting of memory loss. So, the big take away here is: what psychiatric diagnoses can also cause memory loss?

Only major depression. It is uncommon that a medication can cause a mood disorder *and* memory loss.

What is the correct answer?

Major depressive disorder

Remind yourself that this exam is all about probability. Position yourself favorably by considering the probability of a given answer being correct. Using a probabilistic way of thinking can help you to arrive at and feel more confident in your answer. We cannot know everything all the time. Do the best you can.

Question 3

A 38-year-old woman presents to clinic for her routine gynecologic exam. She has a history of major depressive disorder, fibromyalgia, and migraine with aura, but is otherwise healthy. Her medications include duloxetine and topiramate. Family history is negative for ovarian, breast, or colon cancer. She denies vaginal or vulvar itching or pain, dysuria or hematuria, hot flashes or mood swings. The patient does endorse pelvic pain, but only during menstruation. The pain sometimes causes her to call out from work. She denies dyspareunia and has had three male sexual partners over her lifetime. She reports inconsistent condom use and is interested in discussing alternative options for contraception. Her last period was 2 weeks ago, and she menstruates every 27–30 days. She denies heavy bleeding. The patient is well appearing. The abdomen is soft, nontender, without palpable masses on abdominal or bimanual exam. There is no vulvar or vaginal erythema on exam. Cervix is mobile, nontender, and nonfriable. Which of the following is the best type of contraception for this patient?

a. Copper intrauterine device
b. Tubal ligation
c. Combination oral contraceptives
d. Hormonal intrauterine device
e. Barrier method combined with withdrawal

Step 1: Read the last two sentences, then the first two. This includes the question.

This reads:

Cervix is mobile, nontender, and nonfriable. Which of the following is the best type of contraception for this patient?

A 38-year-old woman presents to clinic for her routine gynecologic exam. She has a history of major depressive disorder, fibromyalgia, and migraine with aura, but is otherwise healthy.

What I've learned:

- Mobile, nonfriable, nontender cervix
- 38-year-old woman
- Routine exam
- History of depression, fibromyalgia, migraine with aura

Step 2: Interpret and synthesize the information in the vignette to inform a differential.

Interpretation:

- Normal cervix: Unlikely pelvic inflammatory disease
- Young woman: Less likely malignancy
- Routine exam: Less likely acute concerns
- Medical history: Will likely guide our decision in selecting the best type of contraception

What's our synthesis?

A 38-year-old woman with major depressive disorder, fibromyalgia, and migraine with aura presents for routine exam requesting contraception.

Step 3: Anchor yourself to an answer before reading the answer choices.

As a reminder, the question reads:

Which of the following is the best type of contraception for this patient?

The vignette will likely contain some important information about this patient that will guide us in our decision to choose one option over another. We do not have enough information yet to anchor.

For an average, 38-year-old female patient, oral contraceptives are always a good place to start. They are effective, noninvasive, and typically have minimal side effects.

An intrauterine device (IUD) is a great option for those patients who don't mind a procedure. The IUD can be placed in clinic by a primary clinician or gynecologist and requires no sedation. The IUD itself is quite small, only slightly larger than a quarter (Figure 2-3). The two major classes include hormonal and nonhormonal (copper) IUDs. These devices provide long-lasting protection against pregnancy and their action is local, thereby limiting side effects. The side effect profile varies depending on the class of IUD.

The progestin injection or implant is a less popular option but is still preferred by many patients. Progestin has a less favorable side effect profile compared to combination products. The combination of estrogen and progestin typically helps to control acne and is weight neutral. In comparison, progestin-only products sometimes result in weight gain and worsen acne. And while the progestin-only injections and implant provide longer lasting protection than the pill, they provide less protection than the IUDs.

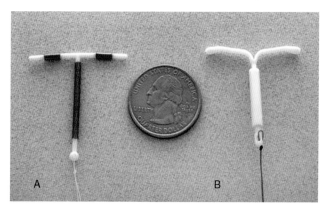

FIGURE 2-3 **Copper and Hormonal Intrauterine Devices.** Intrauterine devices beside a quarter for size comparison. A: Copper intrauterine device. B: Hormonal intrauterine device. (Reproduced with permission from Hoffman BL, Schorge JO, Halvorson LN et al. *Williams Gynecology*, 4th ed. McGraw Hill, 2020.)

We can also consider the test writer's goal in writing this question.

What knowledge is the test writer trying to test?

The test writer's goal is likely to test your knowledge of the individual differences between contraception options and why some contraception is best for or contraindicated in certain individuals over others.

Can you think of some of the unique features of the most common contraceptive options?

Let's review some:

Contraindications for combination oral contraceptives:

- Smoking
- Clot disorder
- Hypertension could be a consideration
- Migraine with aura (higher risk of blood clot)

Benefits to combination oral contraceptives:

- Reduced risk of breast and ovarian cancer
- Regulate menstrual bleeding
- Less heavy, painful menses
- Can skip menstrual bleeding all together

Other contraceptive devices that help with heavy or painful menses:

- Hormonal IUD
- Progesterone injection
- Implant

Hormonal IUD features:

- Need to be able to tolerate the procedure
- Hormonal exposure is primarily local
- Lasts 5 years

Copper IUD features:

- No hormonal exposure
- Can often lead to heavier, more painful menses
- Lasts 10 years

Progesterone injection or implant:

- Unreliable effect on menses
- Easier to remember than a daily pill
- Variable duration of coverage

Based on our list of birth control options and what we know about this scenario so far, we can already rule out combination oral contraceptives as a correct answer. This is because our patient has a history of migraine with aura.

As a good rule of thumb, the contraceptives that have the most significant side effects will be the most heavily tested. Usually, this includes oral contraceptives and their relationship with clot risk, hypertension, migraine with aura, and, less commonly, liver cysts. Another high-yield side effect is the heavier menses associated with copper IUDs.

Even though we still don't have enough information to anchor, we have done enough preparation to move on to the next step.

Step 4: Read the answer choices and try to choose an answer before reading the rest of the vignette, if possible.

As a reminder, the answer choices read:

a. *Copper intrauterine device*
b. *Tubal ligation*
c. *Combination oral contraceptives*
d. *Hormonal intrauterine device*
e. *Barrier method combined with withdrawal*

Let's think through each answer choice:

a. *Copper intrauterine device*: Copper IUD is less popular due to the potential side effects of heavier, more painful menses, as detailed above. Because of these side effects, the copper IUD is avoided in patients with painful or heavy periods, as this has the potential to aggravate their symptoms. This is a good option for patients who do not have significant menstrual symptoms and prefer no hormonal exposure and/or the 10-year coverage.

b. *Tubal ligation*: A tubal ligation is almost never the correct answer on a board exam. Even minimally invasive surgery with a laparoscopic approach carries risk. Non-surgical options, if an option, will almost always be preferred. The test writer would need to provide a big clue supporting this answer choice if it was indeed correct.

c. *Combination oral contraceptives*: We have already thought about the benefits and contraindications for this answer choice. If we remembered that migraine with aura is a contraindication, then we know this isn't the right answer. If we didn't remember, we at least know that we are going to look out for reasons why this would be or would not be the best choice for our patient.

d. *Hormonal intrauterine device*: This is a great option for those who cannot remember to take a pill and/or those who want lighter, less painful menses. The local hormone makes this option safer for those who are at higher risk of blood clots compared to combination oral contraceptives. Because we have the option to choose both a copper or a hormonal IUD, it'll be important to determine what factors in the vignette support the choice of one option versus the other, or neither.

e. *Barrier method combined with withdrawal*: From a medical standpoint, this is never going to be a best option. The other options listed are at least >90% effective with standard use, unlike the barrier method or withdrawal.

Though not an answer choice, a progestin-only pill could be a good option for her. Progestin-only oral contraceptives may be a good option for those who oral contraceptives are contraindicated and prefer to avoid procedures or injections. Side effects include the standard, progestin-only side effects such as acne and weight gain. The drawback of progestin-only pills is that they need to be taken at the same time every day to be effective, whereas the combination pill allows for a less strict schedule. This medication may be "contraindicated" in someone who is described as forgetful or has an unpredictable schedule.

By combining Steps 3 and 4, we can start to anchor on possible answer choices.

What do you think are the most probable answer choices?

The hormonal or copper IUD seem to be the best answer choices based on what we know so far. If we did not remember that combination oral contraceptives are contraindicated in patients with migraine with aura, then this would also be a reasonable consideration.

Now that we have done this work, we can start reading the vignette with the goal of identifying clues that favor the hormonal IUD, the copper IUD, or combination oral contraceptives, if the latter is still a consideration.

Step 5: Read the rest of the vignette.

If you were not able to choose an answer in Step 4, stop reading when you think you know the answer. Then continue reading.

The remainder of the vignette reads:

Her medications include duloxetine and topiramate. Family history is negative for ovarian, breast, or colon cancer. She denies vaginal or vulvar itching or pain, dysuria or hematuria, hot flashes or mood swings. The patient does endorse pelvic pain, but only during menstruation. The pain sometimes causes her to call out from work. She denies dyspareunia, and has had three male sexual partners over her lifetime. She reports inconsistent condom use and is interested in discussing alternative options for contraception. Her last period was 2 weeks ago, and she menstruates every 27–30 days. She denies heavy bleeding. The patient is well appearing. The abdomen is soft, nontender, without palpable masses on abdominal or bimanual exam. There is no vulvar or vaginal erythema on exam.

Before we read the vignette together, I'd like to introduce another strategy. We can call it "Useful, Not Useful, or Trap." This strategy is just as it sounds. After reading a sentence, consider; Is this sentence useful, not useful, or a trap? This strategy is discussed in more detail in Chapter 4 and is used throughout this text.

By practicing the strategy of "Useful, Not Useful, or Trap," we can become a better test taker by thinking more like a test writer.

Let's start with a useful sentence. A useful sentence is one that changes or adds to your working differential. It is a sentence that you need in order to arrive at or solidify your differential and/or answer choice.

A sentence that is not useful should not add much to strengthen your confidence in your answer. Typically, this sentence provides information that is either redundant or superfluous to the vignette. By going through the 5-Step Approach, we are better equipped to identify this type of sentence during our first pass.

Trap sentences can be quite variable. The 5-Step Approach is designed to protect from falling into traps. We will continue to get better at identification of traps with practice.

There are some patterns to identification of traps.

One pattern is that the simplest vignettes tend to be the longest, and the sheer length of the vignette is a trap to lower your confidence level, or to fatigue you, or a combination.

On the same theme, some traps may utilize complex terminology or descriptions designed to lower your confidence. We can try to protect ourselves from such traps by attempting to reword and/or describe those scenarios. We may find through this exercise that the test writer is saying something quite simple.

Let's practice this new strategy:

Her medications include duloxetine and topiramate.

Category: Not useful

Why did the test writer include this?

This information is redundant. We already know that this patient has depression, fibromyalgia, and migraine with aura, which is why she takes these medications. Duloxetine was likely prescribed for both her depression and fibromyalgia and topiramate is likely used to help with migraines. While we should always consider existing medications when prescribing new medications, I am not aware of any medications that would preclude the initiation of an oral contraceptive.

Family history is negative for ovarian, breast, or colon cancer.

Category: Not useful

Why did the test writer include this?

This is filler. Long vignettes test your ability to sift through unimportant information, which is why strategies like this are so important. We need to learn to identify sentences like this quickly and move on.

The preparation we did before reading the vignette should have informed you that family history is irrelevant to answering this question. When we see the phrase "family history," we could even skip to the next sentence.

She denies vaginal or vulvar itching or pain, dysuria or hematuria, hot flashes or mood swings.

Category: Not useful

Why did the test writer include this?

Again, this is filler.

If the patient did have hot flashes and/or mood swings, then we might become more suspicious for menopause. But, based on the answer choices, we should expect that she is still biologically capable of getting pregnant.

The patient does endorse pelvic pain, but only during menstruation. The pain sometimes causes her to call out from work.

Category: Useful

Why did the test writer include this?

This sentence tells us that the patient experiences dysmenorrhea severe enough for her to stay home from work. Whatever contraceptive option we choose should address these symptoms.

She denies dyspareunia, and has had three male sexual partners over her lifetime.

Category: Not useful

Why did the test writer include this?

This is filler.

We already know that we need to choose a contraceptive option that will address her dysmenorrhea. The presence or absence of dyspareunia will not change our decision making, as those contraceptives that alleviate symptoms of dysmenorrhea would also address dyspareunia.

She reports inconsistent condom use and is interested in discussing alternative options for contraception.

Category: Not useful

Why did the test writer include this?

Because of her inconsistent condom use, this sentence might deter us from choosing the barrier method combined with withdrawal. However, we would not have chosen this answer anyway. And, from the question, we already know that we need to select a contraceptive option for her.

Her last period was 2 weeks ago, and she menstruates every 27–30 days.

Category: Not useful

Why did the test writer include this?

Yet again, filler.

She denies heavy bleeding.

Category: Not useful

Why did the test writer include this?

Generally, if a patient experiences heavy bleeding, we would lean towards a hormonal contraceptive and avoid choosing the copper IUD.

In this case, the patient does not complain of heavy bleeding. This means that our choices are not limited by this one symptom. However, we know that she has dysmenorrhea, and that alone will influence our decision. Like dyspareunia, even if she did experience heavy bleeding, our answer would likely not change. Those contraceptive options that help with dysmenorrhea should also help with heavy bleeding.

The patient is well appearing. The abdomen is soft, nontender, without palpable masses on abdominal or bimanual exam. There is no vulvar or vaginal erythema on exam.

Category: Useful

Why did the test writer include this?

I combined these three sentences because they involve the physical exam. While these sentences are not entirely useful, they do tell us some pertinent negatives. Particularly, that this patient has no evidence of a pelvic infection that might explain her dysmenorrhea or preclude IUD placement. An active chlamydia or gonorrhea infection is one of the few contraindications to placing an IUD, though there is no contraindication once the infection has been cleared.

While this patient does have pelvic pain, her pain is cyclical. Cyclical symptoms are largely inconsistent with an infection, and therefore our suspicion for infection should be very low.

After reading through the vignette, we should have hopefully been able to stop and anchor on an answer choice. Whether you were or weren't able to do so, let's go through how we might arrive at an answer choice after completing Step 5.

Though we did not anchor on a specific answer in Step 3, we did narrow our answer choices to the hormonal or copper IUDs, and possibly combination oral contraceptives.

From our preparation, we know that we had to identify factors specific to this patient that would influence us to select one of these options over the others.

What are the two major factors that we should consider in choosing a contraceptive option for this patient?

This patient needs a contraceptive option that:

1. Is not contraindicated in patients with migraine with aura
2. Alleviates symptoms of dysmenorrhea

Based on our work from Step 3, we know that the copper IUD would be a poor choice for this patient given her dysmenorrhea. We also know that oral contraceptives are contraindicated for patients with migraine with aura.

This only leaves the hormonal IUD as the correct answer.

What if you don't remember these facts about contraceptives?

The fact that the test writer included both forms of IUDs might suggest that they want you to differentiate between the two IUDs and select the better of the two options for this patient. When we notice this, we can try to compare both answer choices and try to identify the major difference between them. Sometimes, this can help you to recall information.

For migraine with aura, this is a very specific medical condition for the test writers to mention. Not just migraine, but migraine *with* aura. This should stand out as important, even if you are unsure of the significance.

If you were able to narrow the answer choices to oral contraceptives or hormonal IUD, then you should compare the two to identify the biggest differences. Even with very limited knowledge of the two contraceptives, we should be able to reason through the fact that the hormones from the IUD act locally, whereas oral contraceptives act systemically. We could use this information to consider whether anything in the vignette might suggest a benefit to choosing local rather than systemic effects, or vice versa.

We know the test writer made a point to tell you about a very specific medical condition, and even without knowing the significance, it would not be unreasonable to conclude that local hormone exposure would likely be safer than systemic exposure if there was indeed a contraindication to hormones and migraine with aura.

And, though we classified the sentence about her inconsistent condom use as "not useful," this is another point that might favor IUD placement, as she may forget to take oral contraceptives daily.

While one could argue that patients with dysmenorrhea might be more sensitive to the implantation procedure, the patient does not have pelvic pain consistently, but rather circumstantially. Even if true, this would not be a contraindication in her case.

What is the correct answer?

Hormonal intrauterine device

Even with limited knowledge, we were able to use reasoning skills to arrive at the correct answer.

Remember that we need to try to think of each scenario as a whole, rather than its parts. This is the very basis of the synthesizing that we do in the 5-Step Approach. We need to arrive at an answer that addresses all or almost all the major points in the vignette.

Question 4

A 2-week-old girl presents to the emergency room due to fever and lethargy. The patient was healthy until last night, when she developed a fever and started acting fussier. She was born full-term to a woman who had inconsistent prenatal care and delivered her at home. The mother reveals she has three cats and two dogs at home and drinks milk regularly. She has been refusing feeds since this morning and has not had a wet diaper in 4 hours. Her parents decided to bring her into the emergency room when she became lethargic and difficult to arouse. In the emergency room, her temperature was 38°C. Blood, urine, and CSF samples are obtained. Shortly after the lumbar puncture is performed, the patient experiences a 1-minute, generalized tonic-clonic seizure that responds well to a single dose of lorazepam. The patient appears lethargic on exam and arouses only to painful stimuli. Pupils are equal and reactive to light. Anterior fontanelle is full. There are no rashes present. Cardiac and pulmonary exam are unremarkable. No hepatomegaly on exam. Brain imaging reveals increased attenuation and hemorrhages in the temporal, frontal, and parietal regions.

Vertical transmission of which of the following is the most likely cause of the patient's symptoms?

  a. *Herpes simplex virus*
  b. *Toxoplasma gondii*
  c. *Group B Streptococcus*
  d. *Listeria monocytogenes*
  e. *Cytomegalovirus*

Step 1: Read the last two sentences, then the first two. This includes the question.

This reads:

Brain imaging reveals increased attenuation and hemorrhages in the temporal, frontal, and parietal regions. Vertical transmission of which of the following is the most likely cause of the patient's symptoms?

A 2-week-old girl presents to the emergency room due to fever and lethargy. The patient was healthy until last night, when she developed a fever and started acting fussier.

What I've learned:

  - Attenuation and hemorrhages in temporal, frontal, and parietal regions
  - Vertical transmission of unknown organism
  - 2-week-old girl
  - Fever, lethargy, fussiness
  - Healthy until last night
  - Emergency room visit

Step 2: Interpret and synthesize the information in the vignette to inform a differential.

Interpretation:

  - Attenuation and hemorrhages in temporal, frontal, and parietal regions: Neurologic etiology of seizure
  - Vertical transmission of unknown organism: Important to identify any known in-utero exposures
  - 2-week-old girl: Higher risk of certain organisms and/or illnesses in neonatal period
  - Fever, lethargy, fussiness: CNS signs (fever & lethargy), fever, and neuroimaging in combination are concerning for neurologic infection
  - Healthy until last night: Rapid progression, no apparent congenital abnormalities
  - Emergency department visit: Acute presentation

What's our synthesis?

2-week-old previously healthy girl presenting to the ED with acute onset of fever, lethargy, and fussiness, with changes on brain imaging in the temporal, parietal, and frontal regions, concerning for perinatal infection.

Step 3: Anchor yourself to an answer before reading the answer choices.

As a reminder, the question reads:

Vertical transmission of which of the following is the most likely cause of the patient's symptoms?

We don't have a complete picture of this patient's presentation yet, but we can start to narrow our focus based on what we do know.

What do we know?

We know that this patient was previously healthy, but now has symptoms concerning for a vertically transmitted infection. The fact that she has appeared healthy for the last 2 weeks suggests there are no major congenital abnormalities present, though she has not had any medical evaluation during her lifetime.

What are the most common congenital infections?

The most common congenital infections can be recalled by the TORCH mnemonic.

What does the TORCH mnemonic stand for?

The TORCH mnemonic, or infections, include toxoplasmosis, "other," rubella, CMV, and HSV/HIV. The "other" infections that can be vertically transmitted and are high yield for exams are parvovirus, group B strep (GBS), listeria, syphilis, Zika virus, and hepatitis B.

Are there any distinguishing features in this patient's presentation that we can use to identify the infectious organism?

The main distinguishing feature for this patient is the neurologic changes seen on imaging.

Before we start considering the specific organism that is most likely responsible, let's consider the typical scenario for neonatal fever.

If a neonatal patient presents with fever, regardless of any localizing symptoms, a urinalysis, blood culture, and often cerebral spinal fluid analysis should be obtained to evaluate for the source of infection.

How often is neuroimaging obtained?

Neuroimaging is rarely obtained for neonatal fever, so we must consider why neuroimaging was obtained in this case. When we read the rest of the vignette, we will pay close attention to why neuroimaging was obtained.

While this is easy to gloss over, I encourage you to practice noticing clues like this one. This will help you think like a test writer.

We can also recognize that the neuroimaging results are rather atypical. When we think of neurologic infection, we often will think of meningitis and/or an abscess, which are usually not associated with diffuse, increased attenuation and hemorrhages.

Do you remember which TORCH infections increase neonatal risk of a neurologic infection and/or abnormal findings?

Toxoplasmosis, CMV, HSV, GBS, and listeria are the most common congenital infections that will present with neurologic infections or findings. CMV and toxoplasmosis will more typically result in neurologic findings, rather than a neonatal infection.

What TORCH infections might cause this patient's neuroimaging findings?

While we may not recognize these findings as they relate to a specific exposure, we may be able to recall characteristic neuroimaging findings for other TORCH infections and use this knowledge to get us to the correct answer.

The most classically tested congenital infections that can cause neurologic changes are CMV and toxoplasmosis. These congenital infections present somewhat similarly and are easily confused. This is one of the reasons they are commonly tested.

What are the classic neurologic findings in CMV and toxoplasmosis?

Both congenital infections can cause intracranial calcifications, though the location in the brain differs. For the purposes of this question, this knowledge alone is enough to lower our suspicion for these two infections. We also know that these two congenital exposures are not commonly associated with acute neonatal infection, which should further decrease our suspicion.

What are the most common causes of neonatal meningitis?

The most common causes of neonatal meningitis are GBS, *E. coli*, listeria, and sometimes HSV.

What organism can we eliminate based on the wording of the question?

We know that we are looking for a vertically transmitted infection. This eliminates *E. coli* as a possibility.

Before reading the answer choices, we have already narrowed our differential to GBS, listeria, or HSV meningitis. Plus, we know we should be focused on an organism that could lead to those specific neurologic changes identified on imaging.

Let's review some key features for each of these choices so that we know what to pay attention to when reading the vignette.

GBS:

- Limited prenatal care
- Unknown or positive GBS status
- Penicillin not administered or administered within 2 hours of delivery
- Low CSF glucose, neutrophil predominance

Listeria:

- Limited prenatal care
- Specific mention of dairy products
- Low CSF glucose, neutrophil predominance

HSV:

- Limited prenatal care
- No or late initiation of acyclovir prophylaxis
- Visible genital lesions on maternal exam
- Temporal lobe involvement
- Seizures
- Increased CSF protein and RBCs, with normal glucose and a lymphocyte predominance

While seizure is a commonly described feature of perinatal HSV infection, seizure may result from any meningitis or even fever in general.

One note about listeria; many women consume unpasteurized milk and cheese. But not every woman who consumes unpasteurized milk and cheese will expose their fetus to listeria. Test writers may try to influence your decision by mentioning consumption of these foods. But it is important to pay attention to all the risk factors in the vignette and consider whether another diagnosis is more likely.

In terms of probability alone, listeria is less commonly the correct answer. This may be because there are not a lot of specific features of listeria except for exposure history, and this exposure history is rather common. Given this, we could consider narrowing our answer choices to GBS or HSV.

Step 4: Read the answer choices and try to choose an answer before reading the rest of the vignette, if possible.

As a reminder, the answer choices read:

a. *Herpes simplex virus*
b. *Toxoplasma gondii*
c. *Group B Streptococcus*
d. *Listeria monocytogenes*
e. *Cytomegalovirus*

We already anticipated these answer choices and even narrowed them down to HSV, GBS, and, less likely, listeria. We also have a good road map for when we read the vignette as we evaluate for possible risk factors and other clues. Let's use this as a guide.

Step 5: Read the rest of the vignette.

If you were not able to choose an answer in Step 4, stop reading when you think you know the answer. Then continue reading.

The remainder of the vignette reads:

She was born full-term to a woman who had inconsistent prenatal care and delivered her at home. The mother reveals she has three cats and two dogs at home and drinks milk regularly. She has been refusing feeds since this morning and has not had a wet diaper in 4 hours. Her parents decided to bring her into the emergency room when she became lethargic and difficult to arouse. In the emergency room, her temperature was 38 °C. Blood, urine, and CSF samples are obtained. Shortly after the lumbar puncture is performed, the patient experiences a 1-minute, generalized tonic-clonic seizure that responds well to a single dose of lorazepam. The patient appears lethargic on exam and arouses only to painful stimuli. Pupils are equal and reactive to light. Anterior fontanelle is full. There are no rashes present. Cardiac and pulmonary exam are unremarkable. No hepatomegaly on exam.

Let's practice highlighting the major key features in the vignette that help us to narrow our differential and arrive at the correct answer.

*A 2-week-old girl presents to the emergency room due to fever and lethargy. The patient was healthy until last night, when she developed a **fever** and started acting fussier. She was born full-term to a woman who had **inconsistent prenatal care** and **delivered her at home**. The mother reveals she has **three cats** and two dogs at home and **drinks milk regularly**. She has been refusing feeds since this morning and has not had a wet diaper in 4 hours. Her parents decided to bring her into the emergency room when she became lethargic and difficult to arouse. In the emergency room, her temperature was 38 °C. Blood, urine, and CSF samples are obtained. Shortly after the lumbar puncture is performed, the patient experiences a 1-minute, generalized tonic-clonic **seizure** that responds well to a single dose of lorazepam. The patient appears lethargic on exam and arouses only to painful stimuli. Pupils are equal and reactive to light. Anterior fontanelle is full. There are no rashes present. Cardiac and pulmonary exam are unremarkable. No hepatomegaly on exam. **Brain imaging reveals increased attenuation and hemorrhages in the temporal**, frontal, and parietal **regions**. Vertical transmission of which of the following is the most likely cause of the patient's symptoms?*

Had we not done the preparation in Steps 1–4, we might feel inclined to highlight other parts of the vignette that seem important. Instead, we can remain focused on the key information we need to know to narrow the answer choices further. This should help prevent confusion and panic when reading the vignette.

These are the key facts bolded in the vignette above:

- Inconsistent prenatal care
- Delivered at home
- Three cats
- Drinks milk regularly
- Seizure
- Brain imaging reveals increased attenuation and hemorrhages in the temporal regions

What is the significance of these facts?

Inconsistent prenatal care:

- Increased risk of any vertically transmitted disease due to lack of screening

Delivered her at home:

- Home delivery means that we don't know about exposures at the time of delivery, such as genital lesions or perinatal fevers
- If she was not delivered in a hospital, then she would not have received erythromycin eye ointment, a vitamin K injection, or her hepatitis B vaccine.
- There was no medical evaluation at the time of birth for congenital abnormalities

Three cats:

- Possible toxoplasmosis exposure

Drinks milk regularly:

- Possible listeria exposure

Neonatal seizure:

- Many neurologic processes, such as meningitis, predispose to seizure
- Seizure is a classic presentation of neonatal HSV encephalitis or meningitis for board exams
- Possibly febrile seizure unrelated to the specific infectious organism

Brain imaging reveals increased attenuation and hemorrhages in the temporal regions:

- Narrows differential

Now let's compare these facts from the vignette with the preparation we did in Step 3. Below is the list of major features we generated for GBS, listeria, and HSV combined with the bolded facts from the vignette.

GBS:

- Limited prenatal care: Yes
- Unknown or positive GBS status: Yes
- Penicillin less than 2 hours before delivery: Yes
- Low glucose on CSF, neutrophil predominance: Unknown

Listeria:

- Limited prenatal care: Yes
- Specific mention of dairy products: Yes
- Low glucose on CSF, neutrophil predominance: Unknown

HSV:

- Limited prenatal care: Yes
- No or late initiation of acyclovir prophylaxis: Yes
- Visible genital lesions on exam: Unknown
- Temporal lobe involvement: Yes

- Infant seizures: Yes
- RBC prominence on CSF: Unknown
- High protein, high glucose on CSF, lymphocyte predominance: Unknown

From this list, you can see that this patient has several features from each of these diagnoses. But we must remember that the test writer has to give us some information that specifically differentiates one answer from the rest.

Earlier, we narrowed our differential to GBS or HSV. The test writer did not give us anything specific to rule GBS in or out. By comparison, the temporal lobe involvement and seizure are both suggestive of an HSV central nervous system infection.

What is the correct answer?

Herpes simplex virus

This question is a good example of when exclusion of other answer choices is not the best approach. We cannot exclude listeria or GBS, but we can choose a better answer based on the information provided.

Question 5

The following question is like Question 4, but with modification of the key features.

A 2-week-old girl presents to the emergency room for seizure. The patient was healthy until this morning, when she experienced a 4-minute, generalized tonic-clonic seizure. She was born full-term to a woman who had inconsistent pre-natal care and delivered at home. She has never been seen by a pediatrician. The mother reveals she has three cats and two dogs at home and drinks milk regularly. Vital signs are unremarkable. The patient is lethargic and hypotonic on exam. The patient appears small for age. Length is in the 10th percentile and head circumference is in the 1st percentile. Pupils are equal and reactive to light, but she fails the hearing screen. Cardiac and pulmonary exams are unremarkable. Brain imaging reveals periventricular intracranial calcifications. What is the mode of transmission of the responsible infectious organism?

a. Saliva
b. Cat feces
c. Unpasteurized dairy
d. Mosquito bite

Step 1: Read the last two sentences, then the first two. This includes the question.

This reads:

Brain imaging reveals periventricular intracranial calcifications. What is the mode of transmission of the responsible infectious organism?

A 2-week-old girl presents to the emergency room due to seizure. The patient was healthy until this morning, when she experienced a 4-minute, generalized tonic-clonic seizure.

What I've learned:

- Periventricular intracranial calcifications
- Vertical transmission of unknown organism
- 2-week-old girl
- Seizure
- Healthy until this morning
- Emergency room visit

Though this question is asking about the mode of transmission, it is essentially the same question as the last but with an added step, because, after establishing a diagnosis, we need to determine the mode of transmission for that organism.

Because this question requires you to take an extra step, there is more room for error. Before, we could review the list of possible infectious organisms and narrow our differential using this list. Now, all we have are a list of potential modes of transmissions. This could make it harder to exclude answer choices.

Step 2: Interpret and synthesize the information in the vignette to inform a differential.

Interpretation:

- Periventricular, intracranial calcifications: Likely neurologic etiology for seizure
- Vertical transmission of unknown organism: Important to identify in utero exposures
- 2-week-old girl: Higher risk of certain organisms or illnesses in neonatal period
- Seizure: Consider which TORCH infections increase the risk for seizures, though may represent a febrile seizure
- Healthy until last night: No obvious congenital abnormalities up until this point
- Emergency room visit: Acute and/or severe presentation

What's our synthesis?

2-week-old previously healthy female presenting to the ED with seizure, with periventricular intracranial calcifications seen on imaging, concerning for perinatal infection.

Step 3: Anchor yourself to an answer before reading the answer choices.

As a reminder, the question reads:

What is the mode of transmission of the responsible infectious organism?

Though the question asks about mode of transmission, let's focus first on the infectious organism.

In the last question, we determined that toxoplasmosis, CMV, HSV, GBS, and listeria are the most common congenital infections that will present with neurologic infections or findings. CMV and toxoplasmosis will more typically result in neurologic abnormalities, rather than a neonatal infection.

When reading the vignette, we should pay close attention to features that suggest an active infection like meningitis. If there are no signs of active infection, then the more likely diagnosis would be CMV or toxoplasmosis.

In the last question, we also discussed how both CMV and toxoplasmosis can result in intracranial calcifications, though the location in the brain differs. Given the presence of calcifications in the vignette, we should be most suspicious for toxoplasmosis or CMV. If we see signs of an active infection, then we may need to re-evaluate our assessment of the scenario.

If you don't remember the specific locations of the intracranial calcifications seen in CMV and toxoplasmosis, then hopefully we can use some test-taking skills to help increase the probability of arriving at the correct answer.

It would be helpful if we review the most tested features of CMV and toxoplasmosis. In doing so, we reduce the likelihood of mixing up information when we read the vignette.

It is best to focus on the key characteristics that will help you differentiate one diagnosis from another. For example, CMV and rubella can sometimes be hard to differentiate because of their shared features of hearing loss and "blueberry muffin rash." If we were considering rubella, we would focus on the key features that distinguish the two. In the case of CMV and toxoplasmosis, both are associated with intracranial calcifications, but differ in terms of the distribution of these calcifications.

CMV:

- Hearing loss
- Seizures
- "Blueberry muffin rash" (Figure 2-4)
- Periventricular calcifications (Figure 2-5)
- Transmission via bodily fluids

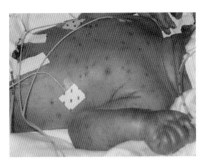

FIGURE 2-4 **"Blueberry Muffin Rash".** "Blueberry muffin rash," or dermal erythropoiesis, is seen here in an infant with congenital CMV. This rash is characterized by violaceous, diffuse, petechial, or purpuric lesions. (Reproduced with permission from Shah SS, Kemper AR, Ratner AJ. *Pediatric Infectious Diseases: Essentials for Practice*, 2nd ed. McGraw Hill, 2019.)

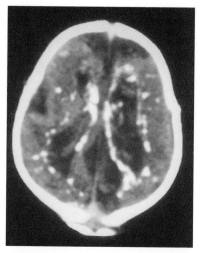

FIGURE 2-5 Intracranial Calcifications Seen in Cytomegalovirus Infection.
Periventricular calcifications are characteristic in cytomegalovirus infection. (Used with permission from Binita R. Shah, MD. From Shah BR, Mahajan P, Amodio J, Lucchesi M. *Atlas of Pediatric Emergency Medicine*, 3rd ed. McGraw Hill, 2019.)

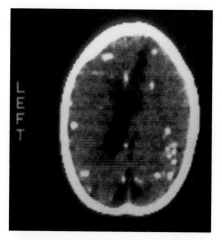

FIGURE 2-6 Intracranial Calcifications Seen in Toxoplasmosis. Diffuse intracranial calcifications are characteristic in congenital toxoplasmosis. (Used with permission from Camille Sabella, MD. From Usatine RP, Sabella C, Smith MA et al. *The Color Atlas of Pediatrics*. McGraw Hill, 2015.)

Toxoplasmosis:

- Hydrocephalus
- Scattered intracranial calcifications (Figure 2-6)
- Chorioretinitis
- Transmission via cat feces or undercooked meat

Step 4: Read the answer choices and try to choose an answer before reading the rest of the vignette, if possible.

As a reminder, the answer choices read:

a. *Saliva*
b. *Cat feces*
c. *Unpasteurized dairy*
d. *Mosquito bite*

What TORCH infections might each of these answer choices represent?

We listed the TORCH infections in the last question. These included toxoplasmosis, "other," rubella, CMV, and HSV/HIV. "Other" infections that can be vertically transmitted and are high yield for exams are parvovirus, GBS, listeria, syphilis, Zika virus, and hepatitis B.

a. Saliva: CMV, rubella, parvovirus
b. Cat feces: Toxoplosmosis
c. Unpasteurized dairy: Listeria
d. Mosquito bite: Zika virus

Because both toxoplasmosis and CMV are possible answer choices, we are unable to further narrow our differential based on the presence of intracranial calcifications alone. While the presence of intracranial calcifications strongly suggests the diagnosis is either toxoplasmosis or CMV, we should always be prepared for the possibility of an alternative diagnosis.

Though it is important to anchor to some degree, we want to avoid excessive or "bad" anchoring.

Step 5: Read the rest of the vignette.

If you were not able to choose an answer in Step 4, stop reading when you think you know the answer. Then continue reading.

The remainder of the vignette reads:

> *She was born full-term to a woman who had inconsistent prenatal care and delivered at home. She has never been seen by a pediatrician. The mother reveals she has three cats and two dogs at home and drinks milk regularly. The patient is lethargic and hypotonic on exam. The patient appears small for age. Length is in the 10th percentile and head circumference is in the 1st percentile. Pupils are equal and reactive to light, but she fails the hearing screen. Cardiac and pulmonary exam are unremarkable.*

Again, I will bold the keywords that are going to help us distinguish between our leading differentials, toxoplasmosis or CMV.

> *A 2-week-old girl presents to the emergency room for **seizure**. The patient was healthy until this morning, when she experienced a 4-minute, generalized*

*tonic-clonic seizure. She was born full-term to a woman who had **inconsistent prenatal care** and **delivered at home**. She has never been seen by a pediatrician. The mother reveals she has **three cats** and two dogs at home and drinks milk regularly. **Vital signs are unremarkable**. The patient is lethargic and hypotonic on exam. The patient appears small for age. **Length is in the 10th percentile and head circumference is in the 1st percentile**. Pupils are equal and reactive to light, but **she fails the hearing screen**. Cardiac and pulmonary exam are unremarkable. Brain imaging reveals **periventricular intracranial calcifications**. What is the mode of transmission of the responsible infectious organism?*

Like the last question, notice how most of this vignette is not bolded.

These are the key facts that I bolded in the vignette above:

- Seizure
- Inconsistent prenatal care
- Delivered at home
- Cats at home
- Vital signs unremarkable
- Length in the 10th percentile, head circumference in the 1st percentile
  Head size is disproportionate to length, suggesting microcephaly
- Fails hearing screen
- Periventricular intracranial calcifications

Why does the test writer highlight that the patient was delivered at home and has never been seen by a pediatrician?

Though we saw some of this in the last question, the fact that this patient has never been seen by a health care professional is far more relevant here. In the last question, the patient was otherwise well appearing outside of her active infection. In this case, the patient is microcephalic with hearing loss. Typically, microcephaly and hearing loss are identified in the hospital after delivery or during the first appointment with their pediatrician.

Before we finished reading the vignette, we were paying special attention to toxoplasmosis or CMV. This is because they are both associated with intracranial calcifications.

Now that we have read the entire vignette, should we consider diagnoses other than toxoplasmosis or CMV?

In the absence of signs or symptoms that suggest an active infection and/or another diagnoses, we can feel confident that the answer is one of these two diagnoses.

Now let's compare these new facts we gathered from the vignette with the preparation we did in Step 3. Here is the list of major features we generated for toxoplasmosis and CMV combined with the additional information we gleaned from reading the remainder of the vignette.

CMV:

- Hearing loss: Yes
- Seizures: Yes
- "Blueberry muffin" rash: No
- Intracranial calcifications: Yes
- Transmission via bodily fluids: Exposure unknown

Toxoplasmosis:

- Hydrocephalus: No
- Intracranial calcifications: Yes
- Chorioretinitis: No
- Transmission via cat feces or undercooked meat: Exposure risk present

Does an exposure risk need to be present to consider a diagnosis?

Not necessarily.

However, if this patient had no known exposures to toxoplasmosis, then the likelihood of this patient having congenital toxoplasmosis would be far less likely.

Perinatal CMV, on the other hand, would not necessarily be associated with a specific exposure. The mother may have had typical cold symptoms or may have been asymptomatic.

By reviewing the list above, we can see that there are more features that favor the diagnosis of CMV over toxoplasmosis. While seizure in the context of fever was of little relevance in the last question, the presence of seizure in the absence of fever has helped us to favor a diagnosis of CMV.

What about microcephaly?

Microcephaly as it relates to CMV is not commonly tested. While microcephaly can occur in both congenital CMV and toxoplasmosis, toxoplasmosis is more likely to present as macrocephaly than microcephaly on board exams.

Why is toxoplasmosis more commonly associated with macrocephaly?

This is because macrocephaly can suggest the presence of hydrocephalus, a key feature of toxoplasmosis and commonly tested on board exams.

While Zika virus is associated with microcephaly (Figure 2-7), there was no other information or exposure history in the vignette to suggest Zika virus.

Notice how we were able to arrive at an answer without remembering the typical location of intracranial calcifications for CMV and toxoplasmosis. Had we remembered that periventricular calcifications are a classic finding in CMV, then we could have answered the question after Step 1.

From Step 4, we know the modes of transmission for the different TORCH infections, so we are ready to go ahead and select an answer choice.

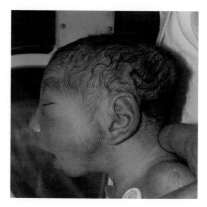

FIGURE 2-7 Newborn with Microcephaly. (Reproduced with permission from Timor-Tritsch IE, Monteagudo A, Pilu G, Malinger G. *Ultrasonography of the Prenatal Brain*, 3rd ed. McGraw Hill, 2012.)

What is the correct answer?

Saliva

Keep in mind that memory can fail you. This is why I recommend against relying on memorization. Always read each vignette with an open mind to ensure you are not mixing up facts. You can always read the vignette with less time and energy than you would have normally just to confirm that your suspicions are correct.

Conclusion

After reading through the examples in this chapter, you may feel overwhelmed. You may doubt that you will have time on an exam to go through all these steps. I want to assure you that, with practice, this process will become fast and feel like second nature to you.

Many students who I have worked with have been resistant to changing their approach at first. Sometimes this is because it has felt too foreign to them. Or maybe because it doesn't make as much sense to them as their old approach. But that approach hasn't been working. And eventually, this new approach should click.

When I first started taking tennis lessons, hitting the ball over the net did not come naturally to me. But I had been playing tennis with friends for a long time, albeit poorly, and had grown used to the way I had been holding my racket. When my coach advised me to change my grip, I was highly resistant. It felt totally unnatural. I thought to myself, "How could anyone hold a racket like this?" But after a few lessons, despite the discomfort, I grew used to this approach and became a better tennis player.

Adopting this new test-taking approach might feel like my experience with tennis. Even if it feels uncomfortable at first, I encourage you to stick with it and keep practicing.

Because you have chosen to read this book, it is safe to assume that your old approach has not been working well for you. So regardless of whether you choose to adopt my 5-Step Approach or an adaptation, make sure to establish a consistent approach to answering questions and rely on this for every question. This consistency will become essential for your test-taking skills toolkit. This will take time at first, and it does not happen overnight, but it will be worth it.

SUMMARY

1. Read the last two sentences, then the first two. This includes the question.
2. Interpret and synthesize the information in the vignette to inform a differential.
3. Anchor yourself to an answer before reading the answer choices.
4. Read the answer choices and try to choose an answer before reading the rest of the vignette, if possible.
5. Read the rest of the vignette.

3

Reasoning

INTRODUCTION

What exactly is reasoning?

Merriam-Webster defines reasoning as "the power of comprehending, infer-ring, or thinking, especially in orderly rational ways."

If that's reasoning, then what is clinical reasoning?

The definition for clinical reasoning is not so clear. In the literature, the defini-tion often extends beyond a sentence to a paragraph or two.

Put simply, clinical reasoning involves the integration of knowledge and experi-ence to reach a diagnosis or develop a treatment plan.

Clinical reasoning is a key factor in what distinguishes an electronic diagnostic tool from a human physician. Arriving at the correct diagnosis or treatment plan is not like a recipe, where symptoms are inputted and out pops an answer. Whether you are reading a patient presentation in a vignette or encountering a live patient, the sum is greater than its parts, and we need to rely on our ability to reason in order to arrive consistently at the correct conclusion.

One of my favorite quotes on this subject reads:

> *"While reasoning errors can coexist with medical knowledge problems, there exists a misconception that clinical reasoning errors are driven by a lack of medical knowledge rather than an inability to apply that knowl-edge in clinical practice."*[1]

The most common problem I see with my students is that they have a lot of medical knowledge but have no idea what to do with it. It is as though someone wrote every fact from First Aid down on various notecards and mixed them up in a bowl. Sometimes they could state a few correct facts, but even when they did, they had no idea how to apply them. And they had no idea how to learn to apply them.

I challenge my students to understand the pathophysiology behind every vignette or clinical scenario. And while it may feel as though you could memorize 50 Anki cards in the time it takes to understand the pathophysiology behind a single concept, I guarantee that your time will be better spent this way. Your understanding of pathophysiology will long outlast any facts you memorize.

When I used to study for exams in college, I relied heavily on memorization. I had stacks of hundreds of notecards in my backpack at all times. This worked great for courses like Biology or Genetics, where I had to memorize hundreds of facts and select the right answer from straightforward multiple-choice questions. But I never used notecards to study for my Physics or Calculus exams. Why? Because these courses rely on your ability to reason through complex problems. What good does memorizing a formula do if you don't know how to apply it?

The following scenario is an example of how medical knowledge and application is much more like Physics than Biology.

In Neurology, a commonly tested concept is the difference between peripheral and central innervation. A particularly challenging aspect to this concept involves understanding the innervation of the face and how a loss-of-function lesion either centrally or peripherally will affect facial movements (Figure 3-1).

Imagine a patient presents with paralysis of the entire left side of their face.

If I asked whether this patient had a peripheral or a central loss-of-function lesion, how sure would you be of your answer?

When you rely on memory, it is hard to feel confident in your answer. But if you are able to use reason, you are likely to be much more assured.

Someone who reasons through their answer can explain why their answer is correct. Someone who relies on memorization cannot.

Years ago, I reviewed this scenario with one of my students who relied heavily on memorization. She often mixed up facts and struggled to understand how to apply the information she had memorized to novel scenarios on exam day.

During one of our sessions, I asked her, "If a patient presents with paralysis of the entire left side of their face, would you diagnose them with a central, or a peripheral, loss-of-function lesion?"

She answered the question incorrectly. But even so, she answered it with a vague sense of certainty.

When I tutor students, I always ask them how sure they are of their answer. This is a strategy you can use while you study or sit for your exams. Assessing

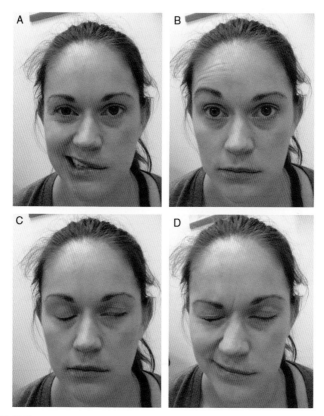

FIGURE 3-1 **Left-Sided Paralysis of the Upper and Lower Face.** A: When the patient attempts to smile, there is no movement on the left side of both the upper and lower face. B: When the patient lifts her eyebrows, only the right eyebrow lifts. C: With gentle attempted eye closure, she is not able to fully close the left eye. D: With more forceful attempted eye closure, she can close both eyes, but there is weakness on the left. (Reproduced with permission from Berkowitz AL. *Clinical Neurology and Neuroanatomy: A Localization-Based Approach.* McGraw Hill, 2017.)

your own level of certainty can serve as a checkpoint for when you are tempted to choose the wrong answer for the wrong reasons.

When asked, this student answered that she was pretty sure of her answer. Her confidence was based in her belief that she could visualize the exact page in her First Aid textbook. In fact, this student was so sure of herself that she challenged me when I told her she was incorrect.

We know that memory is unreliable, and this is a perfect example of that.

Instead of relying on memorization, I encouraged her to reason through the problem with me. I first drew a diagram of the neural pathway, starting from the centers in the brain, to the central neuronal pathways, to the peripheral nerves, ending at the face, explaining the pathophysiology in detail:

> *Simply put, there are two areas dedicated to the face on both the left and the right sides of the brain. One area controls the upper face, and the other controls the lower face.*

> *We know that neuronal pathways in the Central Nervous System need to synapse at a nucleus to pass along information to the peripheral nerve pathways in the Peripheral Nervous System. We also know that most pathways cross before synapsing in the Central Nervous System. We would expect that the left upper and left lower areas of the brain send neuronal signals down their central nerve pathways, cross at some point in the brain before synapsing, and then synapse with the right facial peripheral nerve.*

> *But the facial architecture is special, because the central nerves from the parts of the brain that control the upper face arrive at both the left and the right synapses. This means that the upper face has a back-up mechanism in place; if the area that controls the upper face on the right side of the brain malfunctions, then the area that controls the upper face on the left side will still provide innervation to that same synapse on the right side, sending information to the peripheral nerve despite this malfunction. There is no back-up mechanism for the lower face, so either a peripheral or central lesion will result in lower face paralysis.*

> *As long as the peripheral nerve is working, then that signal will get to the face. But if that peripheral nerve is not working, then there is no way that any signal from the central nervous system can get to the face. There is no back-up mechanism for the peripheral nerve* (Figure 3-2).

After this simplified explanation, my student assured me that she understood the concept and felt confident she would answer this question correctly the next time.

But the following week, I asked her again, "If a patient presents with paralysis of the entire left side of their face, would you diagnose them with a central, or a peripheral, loss-of-function lesion?" And again, she answered incorrectly.

Why do you think she answered incorrectly, yet again?

She was still not reasoning through her answer. She insisted that she had the answer memorized and didn't need to reason through it again. Despite reviewing this concept just one week prior, her insistence on relying on memorization continued to lead her to the incorrect answer. It was not until the following week, when she reasoned through the answer, did she answer correctly.

This example should illustrate the unreliability of memorization and the importance of reasoning.

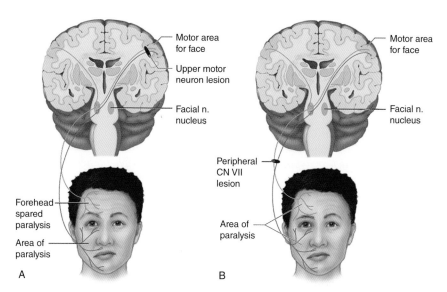

FIGURE 3-2 **Motor Neuropathways for the Upper and Lower Face.** A: Upper motor neuron lesion on the left. No input from the left brain arrives at the facial nucleus. Because the upper face receives input from both sides of the brain, the right brain contributes motor input for the upper face. Paralysis only affects the lower right face. B: Lower motor neuron lesion on the right. Synapse occurs normally at the facial nerve nucleus, but there is damage to the peripheral nerve containing all input for the upper and lower face. There is no redundant input; thus, both the upper and lower face are paralyzed. (Reproduced with permission from Knoop KJ, Stack LB, Storrow AB, Thurman RJ. *The Atlas of Emergency Medicine,* 5th ed. McGraw Hill, 2021.)

Reasoning is probably our most important test-taking skill and will be essential for our future as physicians. While we cannot possibly know everything there is to know about medicine, what we do know can serve as our foundation when we need to reason through novel scenarios and concepts.

Let's focus on our reasoning skills as we work through some practice questions.

Question 1

A 55-year-old woman was brought to the emergency department after a motor vehicle accident. On arrival, she was found to be markedly hypotensive and an aortic dissection was found on imaging. Her blood pressure was stabilized in the emergency department, and she was rushed to the operating room. Following a successful procedure, the patient was admitted for postoperative care. She was encouraged to begin eating solid foods shortly after surgery. On day 3 of her hospital stay, she begins complaining of moderate abdominal pain that is worse after eating. Temperature is 37.5 °C, blood pressure is 110/70 mmHg, pulse is 95/min, and respirations are 18/min. On exam, her abdomen is distended. She has mild tenderness across the upper abdomen. She has foul smelling stool that is tinged with streaks of blood. What is the most likely diagnosis?

   a. Cholecystitis
   b. Postoperative ileus
   c. Colonic ischemia
   d. *C. difficile* infection
   e. *S. aureus* infection
   f. Carbohydrate intolerance

I'd like to demonstrate two different approaches to this question.

The first will involve adding points for and against the answer choices. This approach combines reasoning with the skill of categorizing information as useful or not useful. This strategy was discussed in Chapter 2 and will be discussed in more detail in Chapter 4.

The second approach will require us to reason through the pathophysiology to arrive at the correct answer. If you already know the answer, I encourage you to still walk through these two approaches so that you may use them for future questions.

Let's start with the first approach.

To start, we need to list the key features from the vignette. The major features from this vignette include:

   - 55-year-old woman
   - Status post motor vehicle accident requiring emergency transport
   - Initially hypotensive with traumatic aortic dissection
   - Successful operative repair with normalization of vital signs
   - On day 3, develops abdominal pain, worse after eating
   - Vital signs on day 3 are normal
   - Abdominal exam notable for mild upper abdominal tenderness
   - Foul smelling stool with streaks of blood

We also should characterize each answer choice with a few facts we know about them. Remember from the section on underconfidence that it's okay not to recognize or know much about an answer choice. Focus your energy on those answer choices that are more familiar and work from there.

As a reminder, the answer choices read:

   a. *Cholecystitis*
   b. *Postoperative ileus*
   c. *Colonic ischemia*
   d. *C. difficile infection*
   e. *S. aureus infection*
   f. *Carbohydrate intolerance*

Local signs	Murphy's sign
	Right upper quadrant mass, pain, or tenderness
Systemic signs	Fever
	Elevated C-reactive protein
	Elevated WBC count
Imaging	Imaging findings characteristic of acute cholecystitis
Diagnosis	Suspected: One local sign and one systemic sign
	Definite: One local sign, one systemic sign, and imaging findings of acute cholecystitis
Accuracy	Sensitivity 91.2%, specificity 96.9% for definite diagnosis criteria compared with surgical pathology gold standard

FIGURE 3-3 **Diagnosis of Cholecystitis.** (Reproduced with permission from Tintinalli JE, Ma J, Yealy DM et al. *Tintinalli's Emergency Medicine: A Comprehensive Study Guide*, 9th ed. McGraw Hill, 2020.)

What are some facts that you might associate with each answer choice?

a. *Cholecystitis:* Right upper abdominal pain, sometimes fever, pain associated with meals, risk factors include estrogen, obesity, female (Figure 3-3)

b. *Postoperative ileus:* Slowing of the gut after surgery, looks like constipation

c. *Colonic ischemia:* From hypercoagulable state or organ ischemia due to systemic lack of perfusion, bloody stools, abdominal pain, distention from slowing of the colon

d. *C. difficile infection:* Hospital- or antibiotic-acquired infection, perfuse, foul smelling, watery diarrhea

e. *S. aureus infection:* Common source of infection, such as skin infection, endocarditis, or osteomyelitis

f. *Carbohydrate intolerance:* Foul smelling diarrhea from malabsorption, abdominal distention, and tenderness, not localized, may follow a diarrheal illness

Now let's combine the two lists by taking each answer choice and listing what features from the vignette work in favor of, or against, that answer choice.

a. *Cholecystitis (Figure 3-4):*
   (+) Pain worse after eating
   (+) Female
   (−) Pain not localized to right upper quadrant
   (−) Foul smelling, bloody stool
   (−) Normal vital signs

b. *Postoperative ileus:*
   (+) After surgery
   (+) Abdominal pain
   (−) No constipation
   (−) Presence of blood

c. *Colonic ischemia:*
   (+) Hypotensive state
   (+) Bloody stools
   (+) Abdominal pain
   (+) Distention

d. *C. difficile infection:*
   (+) Hospital exposure
   (+) Foul smelling stool
   (−) No diarrhea
   (−) Presence of blood

e. *S. aureus infection:*
   (+) Possible source from surgery
   (−) Does not explain abdominal symptoms

f. *Carbohydrate intolerance:*
   (+) Foul smelling stool
   (+) Abdominal distention and tenderness
   (−) No clear antecedent
   (−) No diarrhea

The correct answer should be the choice with the most supporting evidence and/ or the choice with the least contradictory evidence.

Let's move on to the second approach. Different approaches will be better depending on the question and the fund of knowledge you have in your artillery. Sometimes we may even combine approaches.

For this approach, we are going to use our knowledge of basic physiology to reason our way to an answer. This is the old-fashioned, original test-taking skill.

How would you describe the context?

In this question, we have a female patient who has suffered a traumatic injury and is subsequently found to have hypotension secondary to an aortic dissection.

How hypotensive do we think this patient was?

Probably *really* hypotensive. One big hint is that she required a large volume of blood transfusions.

Disease	Symptoms	Physical Examination	Ultrasonography	Laboratory Studies
Biliary colic	Postprandial pain, usually <6 h in duration	Afebrile, mild tenderness over gallbladder	Gallstones in gallbladder but no wall thickening, no CBD dilation	Normal WBC count, normal LFT values, normal serum amylase level
Acute cholecystitis	Persistent epigastric or RUQ pain lasting >8 h	May be febrile or afebrile; usually localized gallbladder tenderness	Gallstones in gallbladder; may have pericholecystic fluid; may or may not have CBD dilation	Normal or elevated WBC count; may have normal or mildly elevated LFT values
Chronic cholecystitis	Persistent recurrent RUQ pain	Afebrile; may have localized tenderness over a palpable gallbladder	Stones in gallbladder, thickened gallbladder wall; in advanced cases contracted gallbladder	Normal WBC count; may have mild elevation in LFT values
Choledocholithiasis	Postprandial abdominal pain that improves with fasting	May or may not be clinically jaundiced; nonspecific RUQ abdominal tenderness	Gallstones in gallbladder; CBD usually dilated	Elevation in LFT values; the pattern of elevation is dependent on the chronicity and partial vs. complete obstruction
Biliary pancreatitis	Persistent epigastric and back pain	Epigastric tenderness to deep palpation is present	Gallstones in gallbladder; CBD dilation may occur because of pancreatitis (does not always indicate CBD stones)	Leukocytosis, serum amylase level frequently >1000 U/L, LFT values may be transiently elevated, but persistence may indicate CBD stones

FIGURE 3–4 Comparing Gallbladder Pathologies. (Reproduced with permission from Toy EC, Liu TH, Campbell AR, Palmer BJA. *Case Files: Surgery,* 5th ed. McGraw Hill, 2016.)

What do we know about severe hypotension and its sequelae?

At a very basic level, severe hypotension should cause you to worry about hypo-perfusion. Less blood flow means less oxygen delivery to tissues and organs.

One of the most tested sequelae of systemic hypoperfusion is pre-renal acute kidney injury (AKI). But other organs can also become ischemic if the hypoten-sion is severe enough, including the colon.

If your colon is ischemic, then you may present with symptoms of malabsorp-tion, such as foul-smelling stool and abdominal distention. Ischemia also results in tissue death and sloughing of blood into the stool.

Colonic ischemia could explain the key features we identified in the vignette. But let's reason through the other answer choices before making a final decision.

In a typical scenario, cholecystitis would be our go-to diagnosis. An otherwise healthy female presents to the emergency room with abdominal pain, worse after eating. Majority of the time this is cholecystitis.

But we know this patient developed these symptoms while hospitalized.

What are the chances this patient randomly developed cholecystitis during her admission?

The chances that this patient developed cholecystitis coincidentally are low. If we were to select this answer choice, we should only do so if we had a reasonable explanation for why a motor vehicle accident, aortic dissection, surgery, and/or hypoperfusion might increase the risk of cholecystitis. If there is no reasonable explanation, then this answer choice should be excluded. And, even if there was a reasonable explanation, her lack of fever might suggest against an inflamma-tory etiology such as cholecystitis.

Abdominal pain after surgery is commonly caused by postoperative ileus and looks a lot like constipation. This is essentially a slowing of your colon. We can only con-sider this diagnosis if this can explain all her symptoms and exam findings.

This patient has a few symptoms that would argue against a diagnosis of postoperative ileus. Foul smelling stool is atypical and should raise suspicion for malabsorption. And streaks of blood are concerning for certain infections, inflammation, or ischemia.

While *C. difficile* is an infectious process, the presence of blood is inconsistent with this diagnosis. If the patient had recently been on antibiotics, we might be tempted to consider *C. difficile*, especially given the foul-smelling stool. How-ever, this diagnosis would not be able to explain the whole picture.

If we focus on the foul-smelling stool, carbohydrate intolerance might seem like a likely diagnosis. However, carbohydrate intolerance is not typically acute or triggered by a traumatic accident. While some patients can become temporarily lactose intolerant after a diarrheal illness, we would expect a different time course of symptoms. It's important for us to combine her risk factors with her presentation, because a different set of risk factors might suggest another diagnosis.

Colonic ischemia is the one diagnosis that can be caused by the event leading to her hospitalization and can explain her foul smelling, bloody stool.

What is the correct answer?

Colonic ischemia

Notice how the second approach was very similar to the first approach, but with less structure and a larger emphasis on reasoning through the underlying physiology.

Question 2

A 17-year-old girl is brought to the emergency department by her mother for lethargy. Over the last day, she has become increasingly lethargic. The mother became concerned when her speech became incomprehensible, and she brought her to the emergency department. Her past medical history is notable for hypothyroidism and poorly controlled asthma. She normally uses a daily prednisone inhaler and albuterol as needed, and just completed a 5-day oral prednisone course 3 days ago. Temperature is 37 °C, blood pressure is 95/70 mmHg, pulse is 115/min, and respirations are 30/min. On exam, her mucous membranes are dry. Cardiopulmonary exam is unremarkable except for tachycardia. Laboratory results are as follows:

Sodium 130 mEq/L
Potassium 4.5 mEq/L
Chloride 95 mEq/L
Bicarbonate 13 mEq/L
Glucose 950 mg/dL
Creatinine 1.5 mg/dL
Blood urea nitrogen 35 mEq/L

The patient is started on regular insulin and normal saline in the emergency department. What is the next best step in management?

a. Urinalysis
b. Renal ultrasound
c. Albuterol nebulizer
d. Sodium bicarbonate
e. Intravenous potassium
f. Intravenous dexamethasone
g. No additional intervention

Depending on your level of comfort with this question, it may seem complex at first. Because this question is less straightforward, starting with the second approach from the last question may serve us better. With a less straightforward question, organizing pluses and minuses like we did in the first approach might be harder to do.

As you become more experienced, you can decide which approach works better for the specific question in front of you.

As we reason through this question, using the basic principles of pausing and synthesizing information as discussed in the 5-Step Approach in Chapter 2 will be hugely useful.

Before we read through the vignette, we should review the labs. Strategies for reviewing labs were detailed in Chapter 1. Those strategies will be applied here.

Let's label each lab as normal, high, or low.

Sodium 130 mEq/L—low
Potassium 4.5 mEq/L—normal
Chloride 95 mEq/L—low
Bicarbonate 13 mEq/L—low
Glucose 950 mg/dL—high
Creatinine 1.5 mg/dL—high
Blood urea nitrogen 35 mEq/L—high

We can start by assessing the fluid status of this patient. Recall that the key lab values that help us assess fluid status include sodium, BUN, creatinine, and the BUN/creatinine ratio.

This patient has a low sodium, a high BUN and creatinine, and a BUN/creatinine ratio >20:1.

How do we interpret these lab values as they relate to her volume status?

Her elevated BUN, creatinine, and BUN/creatinine ratio all suggest a pre-renal kidney injury. This suggests that the patient is hypovolemic.

How would we classify this patient's hyponatremia?

This patient has a hypovolemic hyponatremia.

If we move on to her acid-base status, we see that her bicarbonate is low.

Does a low bicarbonate level suggest an acidosis or an alkalosis?

Even though we do not have the carbon dioxide level, we can conclude that this likely represents a metabolic acidosis. While it is possible that this represents a respiratory alkalosis, this diagnosis is highly uncommon in board exams. And if a respiratory alkalosis is present, there will be enough clinical clues in the vignette to make this diagnosis.

Next, assuming she has a metabolic acidosis, let's calculate her anion gap. We can do this by subtracting the chloride and bicarbonate from her sodium level. A normal anion gap is 12, +/− 2, but her anion gap amounts to 22. This is highly elevated.

To summarize, this patient has a hypovolemic hyponatremia and an anion gap acidosis. We should look for clues that will allow us to figure out what from the MUDPILES mnemonic could explain both her hypovolemia and acidosis. We no longer need to think about her hyponatremia, since we know this is likely a result of her hypovolemia.

The next most significant lab value that we have not yet covered is her glucose level, which is also highly elevated. A highly elevated glucose would suggest diabetic ketoacidosis (DKA) or hyperosmolar hyperglycemic state (HHS). However, given that we know this patient has a metabolic anion-gap acidosis, DKA is the more likely diagnosis. This is represented by the "D" in the MUDPILES mnemonic.

Recall that polyuria is a common symptom in undiagnosed diabetes mellitus and DKA. These patients lose a lot of volume from this osmotic diuresis and often present in a state of severe dehydration. This would explain our patient's hypovolemia.

It is important to note that the diagnosis of DKA can explain all her lab abnormalities: her hypovolemic hyponatremia, her anion-gap acidosis, and her hyperglycemia. Because of this, we can feel reasonably confident in our conclusion.

What is the renal pathophysiology behind the osmotic diuresis in diabetes mellitus?

Below a certain threshold, glucose is fully reabsorbed by the kidneys (Figure 3-5). But if serum glucose levels rise too high, then the kidneys will no longer be capable of reabsorbing more glucose and the excess glucose will be lost in the urine. Because glucose is an osmole, free water will follow the excreted glucose. This means that the more glucose is lost in the urine, the more water is lost with it.

This polyuria can often lead to severe dehydration. While patients often complain of increased thirst and polydipsia, their water intake is often not sufficient to negate the loss of water and glucose in the urine.

Based on labs alone, we were able to arrive at a diagnosis before even reading the vignette. Now we are well equipped to read the vignette in a focused manner that will save time and energy and prevent us from falling into test-writer traps.

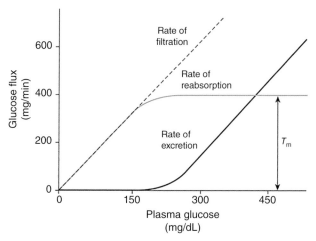

FIGURE 3-5 Glucose Reabsorption and Excretion by the Kidneys. The rates of filtration, reabsorption, and excretion are plotted as a function of plasma glucose concentration. At normal plasma glucose levels, all filtered glucose is reabsorbed, and none is excreted. As plasma glucose levels rise to hyperglycemic range, transport carriers become saturated and are unable to reabsorb all the glucose that flows through the tubule. T_m depicted on this graph refers to the transport rate at saturation, known as the transport maximum, and any glucose filtered in excess of this level is excreted. (Adapted with permission from Eaton DC, Pooler JP. *Vander's Renal Physiology,* 9th ed. McGraw Hill, 2018.)

We are ready to read the question. The question reads:

What is the next best step in management?

We should use our reasoning skills to answer this question. This involves focusing on our knowledge of pathophysiology and applying that knowledge to this clinical scenario.

We already have strong suspicions about a diagnosis, and now we know that our task is to determine the next best step in management. At this point, we should pause to consider the appropriate management for a patient with DKA.

How would you summarize the management of a DKA patient?

At a minimum, this patient will require intravenous (IV) fluids for dehydration and insulin to lower her glucose level. But when we review the answer choices, we do not see IV fluids or insulin listed as possible answer choices. We will need to think of other aspects for DKA management when we read the vignette.

As a reminder, the answer choices read:

a. *Urinalysis*
b. *Renal ultrasound*
c. *Albuterol nebulizer*

d. *Sodium bicarbonate*
e. *Intravenous potassium*
f. *Intravenous dexamethasone*
g. *No additional intervention*

Now we are ready to read the vignette, but let's pause periodically as we do so. This will allow us to continue to reassess our hypothesis as we learn new information.

A 17-year-old girl is brought to the emergency department by her mother for lethargy. Over the last day, she has become increasingly lethargic.

Can DKA explain this patient's lethargy?

Yes. DKA can even lead to coma and death.

Can we explain why DKA might lead to lethargy or coma based on what we know about the pathophysiology?

DKA is a result of insulin deficiency. Insulin is essential for glucose uptake by the tissues. Without insulin, glucose levels increase in the serum, though glucose utilization itself is low. Without the ability to utilize glucose, the body cannot function normally and reacts as though it is starving. Ketones are generated by the liver, which results in ketoacidosis. Acidosis can be dangerous to organs, including the brain.

The combination of severe dehydration, inability to utilize glucose, and acidosis can explain why patients might become lethargic and even comatose.

The mother became concerned when her speech became incomprehensible, and she brought her to the emergency department.

Can DKA explain this patient's incomprehensible speech?

It can. We have just discussed the effects that DKA can have on tissues, including the brain. Worsening mental status because of DKA could lead to this speech impairment.

We should also pause to consider why the test writer decided to present this example of DKA with lethargy and incomprehensible speech, rather than focusing on the more classic signs of polyuria and polydipsia.

Lethargy and speech changes are less common, and therefore more difficult to recognize as DKA. Had we not first reviewed the labs, we may have been thrown off by these symptoms and built an alternative differential for this scenario.

Her past medical history is notable for hypothyroidism and poorly controlled asthma.

Why did the test writer choose these diagnoses as part of her past medical history?

Sometimes, there is a reason why the test writer chooses certain medical conditions. More often it is irrelevant or intended to cloud your understanding of the scenario. This is why it is often useful to ask yourself, "Is this information useful, not useful, or a trap?"

Is there any connection between hypothyroidism, asthma, and diabetes?

Let's start with hypothyroidism. Both hypothyroidism and diabetes mellitus can arise from autoimmune processes. A medical history or family history of any of these diagnoses should increase your suspicion for another. Celiac disease and vitiligo are other examples of these autoimmune diseases that tend to cluster. DKA tends to be more highly associated with type I diabetes, and her history of hypothyroidism might make us feel more confident in our diagnosis.

Is there any connection between diabetes and asthma?

Not that I am aware of.

Can you think of any reason why the test writer chose to list asthma as part of her medical history?

We talked about how past medical history can sometimes serve to confuse and/ or distract the test taker.

How might a past medical history of asthma confuse a test taker in this case?

Consider the fact that this patient has an acid-base disturbance. In the unlikely case that you fail to notice her hyperglycemia, you might misattribute her acid-base disturbance to hyper- or hypoventilation caused by her asthma.

Instead of jumping to conclusions about asthma and breathing irregularities resulting in her acid-base disturbance, we should think through the pathophysiology. We should first recognize that early stages of asthma with hyperventilation should result in a respiratory alkalosis, not an acidosis. Only in late stages of asthma do we see respiratory acidosis from hypoventilation. And, even if respiratory acidosis were present, the bicarbonate would increase, not decrease, in an effort to compensate for the acidosis.

She normally uses a daily prednisone inhaler and albuterol as needed, and just completed a 5-day oral prednisone course 3 days ago.

We should play close attention to anything that happened around the same time as the onset of symptoms. The recent initiation or termination of a medication is likely relevant to her presentation.

Is there a link between steroids and DKA?

Indeed, steroid use can precipitate DKA. But it is important to point out that we do not actually need to know this fact to answer this question. Our focus is on the best next step for management, not what might have precipitated her DKA.

Temperature is 37 °C, blood pressure is 95/70 mmHg, pulse is 115/min, and respirations are 30/min. On exam, her mucous membranes are dry. Cardiopulmonary exam is unremarkable except for tachycardia.

How would you summarize these exam findings?

This patient is afebrile, mildly hypotensive, tachycardic, and tachypneic. She has dry mucous membranes.

Can our diagnosis explain these findings?

Yes! We know that she is dehydrated, which is reflected by her hypotension, tachycardia, and dry mucous membranes (Figure 3-6). We also know that she is acidotic, which is likely reflected by her compensatory tachypnea. Recall that hyperventilation raises the pH, while hypoventilation will decrease the pH.

The patient is started on regular insulin and normal saline in the emergency department.

Signs and Symptoms	Mild (3–5% body weight)	Moderate (5–10% body weight)	Severe (>10% body weight)
Mental status	Alert/restless	Irritable and drowsy	Lethargic
Respirations	Normal	Deep ± rapid	Deep and rapid
Pulse	Normal	Rapid and weak	Weak to absent
Blood pressure	Normal	Normal with orthostasis	Low
Mucous membranes	Moist	Dry	Very dry
Tears	Present	Decreased	Absent
Skin turgor	Pinch and retract	Tenting	Tenting to doughy
Urine output	Normal	Decreased	Absent
Capillary refill	<2 seconds	2–3 seconds	>3 seconds

FIGURE 3-6 Signs and Symptoms of Mild, Moderate, and Severe Dehydration in the Pediatric Patient. There should be no signs or symptoms present in cases of mild dehydration. If any signs or symptoms of dehydration are present, then the dehydration should be classified as moderate or severe. (Reproduced with permission from Sherman SC, Weber JM, Schindlbeck MA, Patwari RG. *Clinical Emergency Medicine.* McGraw Hill, 2014.)

This is the most important information we have received throughout the vignette. In fact, I could argue that there was nothing useful whatsoever in the vignette up until this point. The labs were all we needed to arrive at a diagnosis, and the vignette only served to support our conclusion.

Now we can start to think through the management plan for this patient.

Prior to reading the vignette, we determined that IV fluids would be important for rehydration, and insulin would be important to address her hyperglycemia. Because both were done in the emergency department, we need to consider what else might be important in the management of this patient.

We know that the possibilities are limited by the answer choices, so we can review them to determine if any choice stands out. While you do not need to exclude all the answer choices, reviewing the possibilities provided by the test writer can guide us towards an answer.

The typical way to review answer choices is to consider whether an answer is correct or incorrect. But another useful strategy involves considering why the test writer chose to include each answer choice.

Let's practice this strategy when we review the answer choices.

As a reminder, the answer choices read:

   a. *Urinalysis*
   b. *Renal ultrasound*
   c. *Albuterol nebulizer*
   d. *Sodium bicarbonate*
   e. *Intravenous potassium*
   f. *Intravenous dexamethasone*
   g. *No additional intervention*

Why did the test writer include urinalysis as an answer choice?

Urinalysis can provide information about proteinuria as it relates to glomerulonephritides, ketonuria and glucosuria as it relates to DKA, hematuria as it might relate to renal calculi, and bacteriuria as it relates to infection. Dehydration can also be suggested by a high specific gravity +/− proteinuria.

Starting with infection, while it would be unusual for a young patient to present with altered mental status in the case of a urinary tract infection, an 80-year-old patient might. In fact, altered mental status is often the presenting sign of infection in elderly patients.

If this patient did have an infection, how could we explain some of the other lab abnormalities?

Sepsis and/or dehydration can result in a pre-renal AKI. A build up of lactic acidosis or even mild ketoacidosis from starvation can result in an anion-gap acidosis.

In this case, given the patient's younger age, we should have a low suspicion for a urinary tract infection.

Should we consider the possibility of intrinsic renal pathology?

Though there are some signs of renal pathology, we were able to explain this by the patient's dehydration resulting in AKI. If her BUN/Cr ratio was <20, we might consider a urinalysis and/or renal biopsy to evaluate for diabetic nephropathy or other renal etiologies.

Do we need a urinalysis to help us solidify our diagnosis of DKA?

We don't need a urinalysis to diagnose DKA. While some will obtain serial urinalyses for patients with DKA, this is to ensure their ketonuria clears. This is not relevant for this scenario in the acute phase.

How else could you determine whether urinalysis was a reasonable answer choice?

This patient can be categorized as high acuity. She is lethargic, altered, and severely dehydrated in the emergency room. We first need to stabilize this patient prior to ordering any nonemergent studies. If we were to choose urinalysis, we would have to ensure there are no better answer choices that would help to stabilize the patient.

Why did the test writer include renal ultrasound as an answer choice?

This answer choice alludes to renal pathology. Before a renal ultrasound, we should obtain a urinalysis to evaluate whether there is any evidence of renal pathology beyond a pre-renal AKI. Depending on the urinalysis results, we might later decide to order an ultrasound or even a CT.

Why did the test writer include albuterol nebulizer as an answer choice?

We know this patient has poorly controlled asthma and that she recently completed a steroid course, likely for an exacerbation. Some of her objective findings, including tachypnea and acidosis, may be concerning for a respiratory pathology. Taken all together, asthma exacerbation may seem like a reasonable possibility.

However, notice how our explanation fails to acknowledge important aspects of the vignette. Though she may have had an asthma exacerbation recently, her symptoms should be much improved after completion of steroids. In fact, her symptoms began after completing her steroid course, suggesting her current presentation is unrelated.

The absence of some key features should also deter us from thinking about asthma. Most notably, no wheezes or respiratory distress was appreciated on exam. Absence of these findings would be highly surprising in an asthma exacerbation.

Why did the test writer include sodium bicarbonate as an answer choice?

We can attribute this patient's low bicarbonate to her acidotic state. We would expect the acidosis to correct after correcting her DKA. Bicarbonate could be the correct answer choice if we urgently needed to correct her acidosis.

How would we know whether this patient needs a more urgent intervention for her acid-base imbalance?

If this patient was severely altered or comatose, or there are signs of worsening organ dysfunction, it might be reasonable to consider an additional intervention to expedite the resolution of her acidosis. However, wouldn't sodium bicarbonate serve as only a temporary fix for a problem better solved at the source with insulin?

If we were worried that insulin would not act rapidly enough to correct her acidosis, or that her acidosis was so severe that we needed to initiate an additional therapy or therapies, then we should probably consider an intervention that will have a greater effect than bicarbonate alone. Remember that this patient is actively using up bicarbonate, and any supplemental bicarbonate given will also be rapidly used.

In the case of severe acidosis, dialysis is a consideration.

You may recall the AEIOU mnemonic for scenarios in which you would consider dialysis. The mnemonic stands for acid-base abnormalities, electrolyte abnormalities, intoxication or ingestion, overload (fluid), and uremia (Figure 3-7).

While this patient does have altered mental status and AKI, she does not appear to be rapidly deteriorating and her clinical course has been progressive over several days. Because she is relatively stable, it would be reasonable to wait and see how she responds to the standard-of-care interventions before escalating treatment.

Why did the test writer include intravenous potassium as an answer choice?

If you have been practicing thinking like a test writer, this answer choice should stand out to you. Why?

Because her potassium level is normal. Test writers only include answer choices that are either correct or seem like they could be correct. They would not include an answer that is obviously incorrect.

If her potassium level is normal, isn't intravenous potassium obviously incorrect?

To answer this question, let's consider how potassium is related to diabetes and DKA.

We should start by reviewing the pathophysiology of potassium regulation and the factors that affect potassium levels.

A	Acid–base abnormalities
	Metabolic acidosis is the most common disorder seen and can predispose patients to cardiac arrhythmias.
E	Electrolyte abnormalities
	Hyperkalemia is the most common abnormality seen as the kidneys are responsible for ~95% of the total body elimination. Hyperkalemia can be life threatening, leading to fatal arrhythmias.
I	Intoxication or ingestion
	Whether toxic concentrations are intentional, accidental, or simply a consequence of decreased elimination, renal replacement therapy may be employed to remove water soluble or renally excreted compounds that have a low molecular weight. Volume of distribution and protein binding may not preclude clearance with dialysis under toxic conditions.
O	Overload—fluid overload
	Pulmonary edema is a life-threatening complication of disease (heart failure) or volume resuscitation that can occur quickly.
U	Uremia
	Uremia is a clinical syndrome that occurs due to the accumulation of all of the substances that the body cannot eliminate in severe kidney insufficiency. While all of the toxic substances have not been identified, metabolic wastes, drugs, and other substances may cause symptoms such as intractable nausea/vomiting, pruritus, pericarditis, asterixis, encephalopathy, and seizures. Patients are also at increased bleeding risk due to platelet inhibition.

FIGURE 3-7 **Indications for Renal Replacement Therapy Using the AEIOU Mnemonic.** (Reproduced with permission from Sutton SS. *McGraw Hill's NAPLEX Review Guide*, 4th ed. McGraw Hill, 2021.)

Total body potassium is regulated by the kidneys, but serum potassium is exchanged intracellularly. When we measure potassium levels, we are measuring the intravascular and/or serum potassium.

Let's recall the intracellular transmembrane exchange.

What factors present in the vignette might increase or decrease intravascular and cellular potassium exchange?

In a homeostatic state, we should achieve a relative balance between intravascular and cellular potassium. In this case, we have established that this patient is acidotic. An excess of hydrogen ions drives potassium into the intravascular space in exchange for increased cellular hydrogen ion uptake.

While her potassium appears normal, this value only reflects her serum potassium. If this patient is not in a homeostatic state, then her serum potassium level may not accurately reflect her total body potassium.

Insulin will also drive potassium into the cells. If we suddenly administer a large volume of insulin to control this patient's diabetes, we risk lowering the intravascular potassium levels.

Let's also consider potassium reabsorption in the kidneys.

What mechanisms can you think of that might contribute to excess renal potassium loss?

Like hydrogen, sodium is often transported across the membrane in exchange for potassium, though not always via an antiporter. If this patient is dehydrated, then we would expect the kidneys to reabsorb more sodium and for water to follow. If more sodium is reabsorbed, then we would expect to lose more potassium in the urine in exchange.

Let's reason this through pathophysiology.

We know that this patient is likely secreting increased aldosterone in a state of dehydration.

Can you recall the mechanism of aldosterone?

Aldosterone regulates the transmembrane reabsorption of sodium in the renal-collecting duct. Recall that this will change the total body volume, as water will follow the sodium. At the same time, aldosterone antagonizes the reabsorption of potassium.

We can also recall the uses or side effects of aldosterone antagonists like spironolactone. Spironolactone is often prescribed as a cardioprotective agent and/or diuretic. But the classic teaching is that spironolactone is not a highly effective diuretic.

If spironolactone is not a very effective diuretic, why is it prescribed for patients that require diuresis?

Spironolactone is a potassium-sparing diuretic, whereas the other commonly used diuretics are associated with hypokalemia (Figure 3-8). It is often added to a diuretic regimen to negate potassium-wasting effects of loop diuretics or thiazides.

If we remember that hyperkalemia is a side effect of spironolactone, then we can remember that excess aldosterone may result in hypokalemia.

If we consider the path of potassium from inside the cell, we can follow it out across the transcellular membrane, into the intravascular space, through the glomerulus, and finally into the urine. For this patient, we know that there are a few points along this path where she could be losing excessive potassium. And the administration of insulin will only lead to more intravascular potassium loss.

Given this condition, it seems reasonable to consider that this patient might require administration of intravenous potassium.

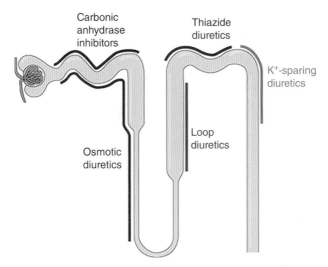

FIGURE 3-8 Sites of Action of Major Classes of Diuretics. Carbonic anhydrase inhibitors like acetazolamide act on the proximal tubule. Thiazides inhibit the Na/Cl cotransporter in the distal tubule. Loop diuretics inhibit the Na/K/Cl cotransporter in the thick ascending limb of the nephron. Aldosterone receptor antagonists like spironolactone are potassium-sparing diuretics that act on the collecting duct of the nephron. (Reproduced with permission from Kibble JD. *The Big Picture Physiology: Medical Course & Step 1 Review*, 2nd ed. McGraw Hill, 2020.)

Why did the test writer include intravenous dexamethasone as an answer choice?

Though a stretch, this answer choice may be tempting for someone who assumes this patient's hypotension and hyponatremia reflect an adrenal crisis precipitated by steroid discontinuation (Figure 3-9). While this might be a tempting conclusion, there is not enough evidence to support this diagnosis. The short duration of steroid exposure makes this theory even less likely.

Is there any relevance of this patient's recent steroid use to our leading diagnosis?

Recent illness and/or steroid use are documented triggers for DKA.

Why did the test writer include no additional intervention as an answer choice?

This is a great answer choice for a test writer to include on an especially tricky question. If you fail to recognize that this patient may need potassium despite a normal serum potassium level, and you recognize that the other answer choices are not correct, then you have the option to choose no additional intervention.

When we don't have this option, it is often easier to realize that we have made a mistake in our reasoning somewhere and select the correct answer choice. If no answer choices seem correct, then we should always re-evaluate the scenario and our thought processes. But, when we have the option to choose no additional intervention, there is no extra hint to tell us we made a misstep somewhere.

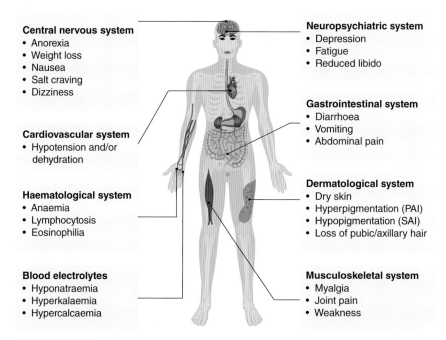

Central nervous system
- Anorexia
- Weight loss
- Nausea
- Salt craving
- Dizziness

Cardiovascular system
- Hypotension and/or
  dehydration

Haematological system
- Anaemia
- Lymphocytosis
- Eosinophilia

Blood electrolytes
- Hyponatraemia
- Hyperkalaemia
- Hypercalcaemia

Neuropsychiatric system
- Depression
- Fatigue
- Reduced libido

Gastrointestinal system
- Diarrhoea
- Vomiting
- Abdominal pain

Dermatological system
- Dry skin
- Hyperpigmentation (PAI)
- Hypopigmentation (SAI)
- Loss of pubic/axillary hair

Musculoskeletal system
- Myalgia
- Joint pain
- Weakness

FIGURE 3-9 **Clinical Features of Adrenal Insufficiency.** (Adapted by permission from Hahner S, Ross RJ, Arlt W et al. Adrenal insufficiency. *Nat Rev Dis Primers.* 2021 Mar 11;7(1):19. doi: 10.1038 / s41572-021-00252-7. Copyright 2021, Springer Nature Limited.)

What is the correct answer?

Intravenous potassium

Though I used many, many pages to answer a single question, we covered an enormous amount of material with just one practice question. And, though it was just one question, we probably covered several questions' worth of information.

We also practiced our ability to tie pieces of information together into a single, larger concept. The more you can do this, the better you will remember, understand, and reason through problems on exam day.

Question 3

A 75-year-old woman is brought to the emergency room by ambulance after she was found partially unconscious on the floor of her living room by her daughter. She had gone to her mother's house to check on her after not hearing from her for 2 days. At that time, the patient's speech was incoherent, and she was not able to stand herself. Her past medical history includes hypertension, hyperlipidemia, diabetes mellitus, and ischemic stroke. She has a 20 pack-year smoking history. Temperature is 38 °C, blood pressure is 100/70 mmHg, pulse is 100/min, and respirations are 22/min. On exam, her eyes open inconsistently and only to voice. Her mucous membranes are dry. Cardiopulmonary exam is unremarkable. Her speech is incomprehensible. She moves only in response to pain. Laboratory results are as follows:

Sodium 125
Potassium 4.5
Chloride 100
Bicarbonate 22
Glucose 850 mg/dL
Creatinine 1.5
Blood urea nitrogen 35

What is the most likely risk factor for her current condition?

   a. Age
   b. Infection
   c. Prior stroke
   d. Smoking history
   e. Dehydration
   f. Renal failure

There are several similarities between this vignette and the last. We can use some of the work that we've already done for this new scenario.

Let's start by organizing the information in the first sentence with the who, what, when, where, and whys. This will provide some structure to how we reason through the vignette.

What are the who, what, when, where, and whys?

Who: 75-year-old woman

What: Partially unconscious

When: Unclear timeline

Where: Neurologic plus other possible system involvement

Why: This is the question we are trying to solve

Can you generate a one-liner from this information?

A 75-year-old woman is brought to the emergency room by ambulance after she was found partially unconscious.

Like the last example, let's start by reading the labs, then the question, followed by the answer choices, and finally the rest of the vignette.

As a reminder, the labs read:

Sodium 125
Potassium 4.5
Chloride 100
Bicarbonate 22
Glucose 850 mg/dL
Creatinine 1.5
Blood urea nitrogen 35

Let's label each lab as normal, high, or low.

Sodium 125—low
Potassium 4.5—normal
Chloride 100—normal
Bicarbonate 22—normal
Glucose 850 mg/dL—high
Creatinine 1.5—high
Blood urea nitrogen 35—high

Let's practice reviewing the labs using a methodological approach, starting with fluid status along with kidney function, then acid-base status, and then electrolytes and glucose.

How do we assess volume status?

We can start with the sodium.

In this case, the sodium is low. Recall both a low and an elevated sodium can suggest dehydration. Dehydration and/or hypovolemia will be the most common cause for a sodium abnormality on board exams.

What do we know about her kidney function?

Her creatinine and BUN are elevated, suggesting renal injury or failure. The BUN/Creatinine ratio is 23.

Does her BUN/Creatinine ratio suggest a pre-renal, intrinsic renal, or post-renal etiology?

A BUN/Creatinine ratio >20 suggests a pre-renal etiology. This is because more BUN is reabsorbed than creatinine as the kidney attempts to reabsorb more volume. Combined with her hyponatremia, it is safe to assume this patient is hypovolemic with a pre-renal AKI as a result.

Now let's assess acid-base status.

The bicarbonate is low-normal.

Should we be concerned for a possible acid-base disturbance?

While borderline normal values can be useful to hint at underlying pathology, the test writer cannot expect test takers to rely on assumptions made from borderline lab values. You will have to be given more concrete information so that you can arrive definitively at an answer.

Finally, we should review the other electrolytes and glucose.

How would you interpret the remaining labs?

While the other electrolytes are in roughly normal range, the glucose is highly elevated.

When we read the vignette, we will now know to pay attention to clues that would suggest a history of diabetes mellitus.

Does this patient have a diagnosis of DKA?

While this scenario appears similar to the last, there are a few key differences, including the fact that this patient is not acidotic. She therefore would not meet the criteria for DKA.

What is a common condition seen in diabetic patients with hyperglycemia without acidosis?

Hyperosmolar hyperglycemic state (HHS).

If we were to describe this patient's lab values, then we would have our diagnosis. Her key lab abnormalities include hyperglycemia and dehydration, which can be attributed to her osmotic diuresis in a hyperosmolar state.

What are some key differences between DKA and HHS?

Besides the acidosis, DKA is more highly associated with type 1 diabetes mellitus and tends to progress more quickly when compared to HHS (Figure 3-10).

Does a diagnosis of HHS explain what we know about the who, what, when, where, and why?

Yes!

This patient was found partially unconscious. We know from the last vignette that altered mental status and coma can occur both with hyperglycemia and acidosis. In this case, only hyperglycemia is present.

Now that we have a good sense of the clinical scenario, let's revisit the question.

As a reminder, the question reads:

What is the most likely risk factor for her current condition?

Without even reading the vignette, we have established a diagnosis of HHS. Now we need to determine the most likely risk factor.

	Mild to Moderate DKA	Severe DKA	HHS
Glycemia	>250 mg/dL		>600 mg/dL
Arterial pH	7.00 to <7.30	<7.00	>7.30
Serum bicarbonate (mEq/L)	10 to <18	<10	>18
Ketonemia/ketonuria	Present	Present	Small
Serum osmolality	Usually <320 mOsm/kg	Variable	>320 mOsm/kg
Anion gap	>10	>12	Variable
Sensorium	Alert to drowsy	Stupor/coma	Stupor/coma

FIGURE 3-10 **Key Features of Diabetic Ketoacidosis (DKA) and Hyperosmolar Hyperglycemic State (HHS).** The key similarity between DKA and HHS is that both states involve dangerously elevated serum glucose levels. The key difference between these states is that DKA involves an anion-gap ketoacidosis. (Reproduced with permission from Farcy DA, Chiu WC, Marshall JP, Osborn TM. *Critical Care Emergency Medicine*, 2nd ed. McGraw Hill, 2017.)

We should review the answer choices and try to answer the question before reading the vignette.

As a reminder, the answer choices read:

a. *Age*
b. *Infection*
c. *Prior stroke*
d. *Smoking history*
e. *Dehydration*
f. *Renal failure*

Do any of the answer choices seem like they might predispose a patient to HHS?

In a perfect world, you would already know what some of the major risk factors for HHS are. If not, we can use our reasoning skills to try and answer this question.

In reviewing the answer choices, you might notice that you can categorize them into two groups. By separating the answer choices into categories, we will have a better idea about what to pay attention to while reading the vignette.

The first group of answer choices, or risk factors, are those that would need to be identified by the test taker based on signs and symptoms described in the passage.

Can you identify these answer choices?

They are:

a. *Infection*
b. *Dehydration*
c. *Renal failure*

The remaining answer choices are those that would need to be explicitly stated by the test writer. If not present, then it is safe to assume that answer choice is incorrect.

Already, we can generate some conclusions about two out of the three answer choices above.

We concluded that the etiology of her AKI is pre-renal based on her BUN/Creatinine ratio in the setting of HHS. Hypovolemia is a common consequence of HHS and provides us with a reasonable explanation for her AKI.

If renal failure and dehydration are both as a result of her HHS, then they are highly unlikely to also be risk factors.

This leaves us only with infection as a possible answer choice from the first group.

When we read the rest of the vignette, we now know to pay attention to any signs and symptoms that suggest an underlying infection.

Now we are ready to read the vignette. Let's practice applying our reasoning skills and knowledge of pathophysiology. Again, let's read in segments and pause to reason through the new pieces of information.

She had gone to her mother's house to check on her after not hearing from her for 2 days.

This sentence provides us with some information about the time frame. We can conclude that she likely became altered over the last 2 days.

At that time, the patient's speech was incoherent, and she was not able to stand herself.

We learn more details about this patient's altered mental status. However, this information does not add much to our clinical picture.

At this point in the vignette, we might have started to develop a differential for her altered mental status. But because of our preparation, we can already attribute her symptoms to HHS. HHS is represented by "insulin" in the AEIOU TIPS mnemonic for altered mental status (Figure 3-11). MOVE STUPID is

A	**Alcohol.** Ethanol. Isopropyl alcohol. Methanol. Concurrent hypoglycemia is common.
	Acid-base and metabolic. Hypotonic and hypertonic dehydration. Hepatic dysfunction, inborn errors of metabolism.
	Arrhythmia/cardiogenic. Stokes-Adams, supraventricular tachycardia, aortic stenosis, heart block, pericardial tamponade.
E	**Encephalopathy.** Reye's syndrome. Parainfectious encephalomyelitis. Autoimmune encephalitis, such as Anti-*N*-methyl-D-aspartate (Anti-NMDA) receptor encephalitis. Posterior reversible encephalopathy syndrome (PRES) may be associated with hypertension, autoimmune disease, and Henoch-Schönlein purpura (HSP).
	Endocrinopathy. Addison's disease can present with AMS or psychosis. Thyrotoxicosis can present with ventricular dysrhythmias. Pheochromocytoma can present with hypertensive encephalopathy.
	Electrolytes. Hypo-/hypernatremia and disorders of calcium, magnesium, and phosphorus can produce AMS.
I	**Insulin.** AMS from hyperglycemia is seen in severe diabetic ketoacidosis, as well as hyperglycemic hyperosmolar syndrome. Hypoglycemia can be the result of many disorders. Irritability, confusion, seizures, and coma can occur with blood glucose levels <40 mg/dL (2.22 mmol/L).
	Intussusception. AMS may be the initial presenting symptom.
O	**Opiates.** Common household exposures are to Lomotil® (diphenoxylate hydrochloride and atropine sulfate), Imodium® (loperamide), diphenoxylate, and dextromethorphan. Clonidine, an α-agonist, can also produce similar symptoms.
	Oxygen. Disorders of airway, breathing, or circulation may adversely affect oxygen delivery to the brain; hypercapnia from primary lung disease or neurologic dysfunction also may result in AMS.
U	**Uremia.** Hemolytic-uremic syndrome can produce AMS in addition to abdominal pain. Thrombocytopenic purpura and hemolytic anemia also can cause AMS. In children with chronic renal failure, neurologic dysfunction may develop secondary to stroke, hypertension, or metabolic derangements.
T	**Trauma.** Hypovolemia or hemorrhage from multisystem trauma may lead to insufficient cerebral perfusion and result in AMS. Consider concussion, hemorrhage, contusion, epidural or subdural hematoma. Consider nonaccidental trauma.
	Tumor. Primary, metastatic, or meningeal leukemic infiltration. Intracerebral tumors commonly produce focal neurologic signs, and posterior fossa tumors typically block the ventricular system and create signs and symptoms of hydrocephalus. Shunt malfunction should be considered among patients with a ventriculoperitoneal shunt for hydrocephalus.
	Thermal. Hypo- or hyperthermia. Progressive hypothermia leads to insidious AMS.

FIGURE 3-11 AEIOU TIPS Mnemonic for Altered Mental Status. (Reproduced with permission from Tintinalli JE, Ma J, Yealy DM et al. *Tintinalli's Emergency Medicine: A Comprehensive Study Guide,* 9th ed. McGraw Hill, 2020.)

another popular mnemonic for remembering common causes of altered mental status (Figure 3-12).

Her past medical history includes hypertension, hyperlipidemia, diabetes mellitus, and ischemic stroke.

I	**Infection.** Bacterial meningitis, encephalitis, and brain abscess usually present with fevers. Brain abscess is characterized by fever and headache before AMS changes. Presenting symptoms also include generalized or focal seizures. Any systemic infection associated with vasculitis or shock may lead to AMS secondary to cerebral hypoperfusion. **Intracerebral vascular disorders.** Subarachnoid, intracerebral, or intraventricular hemorrhages can be seen with trauma, ruptured aneurysm, or arteriovenous malformations. Venous thrombosis can follow severe dehydration or pyogenic infection of the mastoid, orbit, middle ear, or sinuses. Arterial thrombosis is uncommon in children, except in those with homocystinuria. Intracerebral and intraventricular hemorrhages may follow birth asphyxia or trauma in neonates, but in older children, they may signify a congenital or acquired coagulopathy. Cerebral emboli from bacterial endocarditis may cause AMS. Acute confusional migraine may be associated with profound alterations in consciousness. Children with sickle cell anemia can develop cerebral thrombosis, status epilepticus, and coma.
P	**Psychogenic.** Characterized by decreased responsiveness with normal neurologic examination including oculovestibular reflexes. Psychogenic unresponsiveness may be a conversion reaction, an adjustment reaction, a panic state, or malingering. **Poisoning/ingestion.** Drugs, toxins, or illicit substances can be ingested by accident, through neglect or abuse, or in a suicidal gesture. Intentional ingestion of recreational drugs, including synthetic cannabinoids, may be considered.
S	**Seizure.** Generalized motor seizures and absence status epilepticus are often associated with prolonged unresponsiveness in children. In a child with a history of seizures who presents with AMS, consider nonconvulsive status epilepticus. Febrile seizures are seen in children aged 6 months to 6 years.

FIGURE 3-11 (*Continued*)

Altered Mental Status Differential Diagnosis
MOVE STUPID

Metabolic: B12 or thiamine deficiency, serotonin syndrome

Oxygen: Hypoxemia (pulmonary, cardiac, anemia)

Vascular: Hypertensive emergency, ischemic/hemorrhagic CVA, Vasculitis, Myocardial Infarction

Electrolyte and **E**ndocrine

Seizure: Status epilepticus, postictal state

Tumor, **T**rauma, **T**emperature, **T**oxins

Uremia: Renal or hepatic dysfunction with hepatic encephalopathy

Psychiatric

Infection

Drugs: Including withdrawal
• (Anticholinergic, TCAs, SSRIs, BZDs, barbituates, alcohol)

FIGURE 3-12 MOVE STUPID Mnemonic for Altered Mental Status. (Reproduced with permission from Kaufman MS, Ganti L, Chang D, Mena Lora AJ. *First Aid for the Medicine Clerkship*, 4th ed. McGraw Hill, 2021.)

Let's consider whether any of these diagnoses change our working model.

We already suspected that this patient had a history of diabetes mellitus. This history should increase our confidence in our diagnosis. Without this history, we would have had to reconsider our diagnosis of HHS. HHS in an elderly patient without any known history of diabetes mellitus would be surprising, though not impossible.

The other important part of her medical history to highlight is her history of ischemic stroke. This is because prior stroke is listed as one of the answer choices.

Why would a prior stroke predispose you to HHS later?

It wouldn't.

Why did the test writers include this option?

The vignette starts by describing neurologic symptoms as the chief complaint. Given this, the "prior stroke" answer choice becomes more appealing. The focus of neurologic symptoms early in the vignette can make you vulnerable to anchoring on a solely neurologic process. One could argue that the patient suffered another stroke over the past few days, which seems more plausible given her risk factors. She may have become dehydrated due to altered mental status from the stroke, and this dehydration would explain most of her lab abnormalities. However, this theory ignores a significant lab finding: her profound hyperglycemia.

We need to try to arrive at a conclusion that explains the whole picture. A stroke doesn't fit.

She has a 20 pack-year smoking history.

We already expected the vignette to mention a smoking history since this was listed as one of the possible answer choices. If a smoking history was not mentioned in the vignette, then this answer choice could be easily excluded. This would be too easy from a test-writer perspective.

Why did the test writer include smoking history as an answer choice?

If you concluded that this patient's current presentation was consistent with a stroke, then you might decide that this positive smoking history is her biggest risk factor.

Are there any other risk factors for stroke listed as possible answer choices?

Age, prior stroke history, and smoking history are all risk factors for stroke. Other risk factors for stroke are included in Figure 3-13.

Based on our earlier reasoning, we can eliminate the answer choices that represent risk factors for stroke but not for HHS. These include age, prior stroke history, and smoking history.

Recall that the answer choices we just eliminated make up one of the groups of answer choices. Earlier, we had eliminated dehydration and renal failure

	Ischemic stroke	Intracerebral hemorrhage
Nonmodifiable risk factors		
Advanced age	+	+
Family history of stroke	+	
Nonwhite race	+	+
Modifiable risk factors		
Vascular		
Hypertension (systolic >140 or diastolic >90 mmHg)	+	+
Asymptomatic carotid stenosis (70–99% decrease in diameter)	+	
Peripheral artery disease	+	
Cardiac		
Atrial fibrillation or cardiopathy	+	
Congestive heart failure	+	
Coronary artery disease	+	
Endocrine		
Diabetes mellitus	+	
Postmenopausal estrogen therapy	+	
Oral contraceptive use	+	
Metabolic		
Dyslipidemia		
High total serum cholesterol	+	
Low HDL cholesterol (<40 mg/dL)	+	
Abdominal adiposity	+	+
Lifestyle		
Physical inactivity	+	
Cigarette smoking	+	+
High salt, low fruit, & vegetable diet	+	+
Heavy alcohol use	+	+
Obstructive sleep apnea	+	

FIGURE 3-13 Modifiable and Nonmodifiable Risk Factors for Ischemic and Hemorrhagic Stroke. Modifiable risk factors are those that can be targeted by the patient and clinician. Nonmodifiable risk factors include age, gender, race, and family history. (Reproduced with permission from Greenberg DA, Aminoff MJ, Simon RP. *Clinical Neurology,* 11th ed. McGraw Hill, 2021.)

from the other group. This means that we are only left with infection as a likely answer choice.

We should still identify support in the vignette for this answer choice before moving on. This will help us identify any errors we may have made while reasoning through this question. Think of this like checking our work. If there is no evidence that supports a precipitating infection, this might suggest that we missed an important piece of information. We would have to re-evaluate our reasoning.

Temperature is 38 °C, blood pressure is 100/70 mmHg, pulse is 100/min, and respirations are 22/min.

Vital signs are most notable for a fever, low-grade hypotension, and tachycardia.

Our working theory is that this patient had an infection that precipitated her HHS. But we have not yet identified any specific signs of infection until now. Her elevated temperature supports our conclusion, though we do not know the source of her suspected infection.

But how do we explain her hypotension and tachycardia?

We could attribute her hypotension and tachycardia to hypovolemia or sepsis. Both possibilities are consistent with the conclusions we have made.

On exam, her eyes open inconsistently and only to voice. Her mucous membranes are dry. Cardiopulmonary exam is unremarkable. Her speech is incomprehensible. She moves only in response to pain.

These exam findings further support what we already know. They do not add to or change any of our conclusions.

Had the examiner noted rhonchi or diminished breath sounds suggesting pneumonia, we might feel more assured that this patient has an infection. But the absence of these exam findings does not preclude an infection.

Do her neurologic symptoms suggest meningitis?

Meningitis is uncommon in this population. Urinary tract infections and pneumonia are more common.

We know from the last question that it is common for sepsis to present with altered mental status in elderly patients. This is a better explanation for her neurologic symptoms.

In reasoning through the physical exam findings, we should also pay attention to the information that the test writer chose *not* to include.

If the test writer had expected us to diagnose a stroke, shouldn't they have included more information about the neurologic exam?

More than likely, we would see mention of a more extensive neurologic exam, even if findings were normal, such as pupillary reflexes, extraocular movements, strength, sensation, or reflexes.

The test writer should always give you enough information to assure you of the correct answer. Test questions cannot be overly vague. You should never have to come up with an elaborate story or explanation for your answer choice.

If you are still not 100% sure in your answer choice at this point, try to consider the purpose of this question from the perspective of the test writer.

Recall that questions are more likely to test high-yield concepts, more dangerous diagnoses, and conditions with highly testable pathophysiology.

Does it seem plausible that this question is designed to test whether we can identify subtle signs of infection and recognize infection as a risk factor for HHS?

Identification and management of HHS are relatively straightforward. Additionally, HHS is often a less emergent presentation because of the more insidious time course. For these reasons, we can expect HHS to be a less heavily tested concept. In comparison, DKA is often the first presenting symptom of patients with diabetes, presents more acutely, and is complicated by acidosis and hypokalemia. Because of this, we can see why DKA might be more heavily tested.

Identification of sepsis, on the other hand, is very high yield. Sepsis is far more dangerous for patients who are very young and very old, and these are the patients that tend to have subtler symptoms. It seems likely that the test writer wanted us to demonstrate an ability to recognize a subtle presentation of sepsis and identify this as a risk factor for HHS.

What is the correct answer?

Infection

Now that we have answered the question, we should practice summarizing the scenario. This exercise will help prove that we had a strong grasp of the scenario and the reasons behind the answer we chose and will serve to reinforce everything we have learned.

How would you summarize this scenario into one cohesive story?

The summary should read something like this:

> *We have an elderly female with a past medical history notable for diabetes mellitus who was found obtunded by her daughter after she had not heard from her for 2 days. She was found to be septic upon arrival to the emergency room with vitals consistent with fever, tachycardia, hypotension, and tachypnea, though a source was not identified. Her exam was only notable for altered mental status without focal neurologic signs. Labs were concerning for hyperosmotic, hyperglycemic syndrome, with an elevated glucose >600 and no evidence of ketoacidosis. There was evidence of dehydration from her labs as well, including a mild hyponatremia and a pre-renal acute kidney injury, likely secondary to her hyperglycemia and*

possibly exacerbated by prolonged altered mental status and decreased intake.

Did we have to diagnose HHS to answer this question?

No. Much of our reasoning that led us to choose infection as the answer choice was not based on the HHS diagnosis, so we could still feel confident in our answer choice even if we did not feel confident in our HHS diagnosis. We do not always need to know everything about the vignette to feel confident and/or answer a question correctly.

SUMMARY

1. Clinical reasoning involves the integration of knowledge and experience to reach a conclusion.
2. Reasoning requires an understanding of pathophysiology.
3. Be wary of any information that is not supported by your answer choice.
4. Think like a test writer and question why certain information was included in the vignette.
5. Remember that questions are more likely to test more dangerous conditions and/or those with highly testable pathophysiology.
6. Practice summarizing each scenario as one cohesive story that supports your conclusion.

REFERENCE

1. Guerrasio J, Aagaard EM. Methods and outcomes for the remediation of clinical reasoning. *J Gen Intern Med.* 2014;29(12):1607-14. doi:10.1007/s11606-014-2955-1

Categorizing Information & Illness Scripts

4

INTRODUCTION

We as human beings are constantly categorizing information in our surroundings as important or unimportant. Otherwise, the world around us would be an overwhelming immersion of sensory activation. The same is true for standardized exams and clinical practice.

When we begin a patient encounter, our first job is to filter out the important from the unimportant. And what is important may change for every encounter, making this all the more challenging.

The first time I learned this lesson was when I worked as a medical scribe for an orthopedic surgeon. I followed him into patient rooms and wrote patient notes for the electronic medical record. Initially, I thought I would serve as no more than a glorified transcription service. But when I started my training, I realized that my job, unlike a transcription service, required me to document only the important information. This meant that I had to know how to determine what was important.

The problem is, how do we know what information is important?

What's important changes based on the scenario. So, the first step to identifying important information is to understand the scenario in front of you.

From a test-taking perspective, this mimics when we start with the question and answer choices before reading the vignette. This shapes our idea about the kind of information that will be important to pay attention to. Without this primer, we would have a much more difficult time knowing what is and what isn't important.

As we develop our knowledge base, patterns start to emerge. These patterns eventually evolve into illness scripts, and these illness scripts help us to more quickly identify what is important.

What are illness scripts?

An illness script represents our knowledge about a disease in the form of an organized summary (Figure 4-1). This might include pathophysiology, demographics, common signs and symptoms, time course, diagnostics, and treatment. This framework allows us to easily organize new information to determine the likelihood of a disease and disease management.

Imagine illness scripts are each like a fingerprint. When your brain recognizes information presented in certain combinations, it alerts you of a partial or complete match.

Key Risk Factors	Pathophysiology	Clinical Presentation	Diagnosis
• Usually 1-3 mo old infants • Rare after 12 wks of age • 4:1-6:1 male:female • First born son • Maternal smoking increases the risk	• Pyloric muscular hypertrophy • Pyloric canal narrows • Near-complete obstruction	• Nonbilious projective vomiting • Infant demands to be refed soon afterwards • No diarrhea • Severe weight loss • Emaciated with "olive-like" mass on abdominal exam • Hypochloremic metabolic alkalosis • Hypokalemia	• Pyloric stenosis
• Usually idiopathic • Common disorder among adults • More frequent in women • Involved in activities that involve flexing or extending of wrist repeatedly (e.g., typing a book chapter)	• Repetitive actions of the hand or wrist • Increased pressure in the intracarpal canal • Median nerve compression • Ischemia and mechanical disruption of nerve	• Pain and parasthesia in the medial nerve distribution • Worse at night • Changes in hand posture or shaking the hand mitigates symptoms • + Phalen maneuver and Tinel test	• Carpal tunnel syndrome
• Uncommon event • Most common predisposing factor is hypertension • Typically occurs in 60- to 80-y-old men	• Tear in the aortic intima • Degeneration of the aortic media • Hemorrhage into the media • Creation of a false lumen • Propagation of dissection both distal and proximal to initial tear involving branch vessels, aortic valve, and/or pericardial space • Ischemia, aoritic regurgitation, and/or cardiac tamponade	• Severe, "tearing" chest pain radiating to the back • Blood pressure not equal in both arms • Widened mediastinum on chest radiography • Acute hemodynamic compromise	• Aortic dissection
• Most common indication for emergent abdominal surgery in childhood • More common in older children and adolescents • More common in boys	• Obstruction of the vestigial vermiform appendix • Inflammation of the appendiceal wall • Localized ischemia, perforation, and the development of a contained abscess or generalized appendicitis	• Abdominal pain, typically beginning in the periumbilical region and migrating to the right lower quadrant • Anorexia • Nausea or vomiting • Low-grade fever • Peritoneal signs on abdominal examination • +McBurney's point tenderness, Rovsing's sign, iliopsoas sign, and/or obturator sign • Mild leukocytosis	• Acute appendicitis in children
• Most common cause of acute abdomen • Occurs most frequently in second and third decades of life • 1.4:1 male:female	• Obstruction of the vestigial vermiform appendix • Inflammation of the appendiceal wall • Localized ischemia, perforation, and the development of a contained abscess or generalized appendicitis	• Abdominal pain, typically right lower quadrant • Anorexia • Nausea or vomiting • Low-grade fever • Peritoneal signs on abdominal examination • +McBurney's point tenderness, Rovsing's sign, psoas sign, and/or obturator sign	• Acute appendicitis in adults

FIGURE 4-1 **Examples of Illness Scripts.** (Reproduced with permission from McKean SC, Ross JJ, Dressler DD, Scheurer DB. *Principles and Practice of Hospital Medicine*, 2nd ed. McGraw Hill, 2017.)

Let's work through a brief example.

Consider a 50-year-old man with a cough.

What is the most likely diagnosis?

Without more information, there are too many possibilities.

Imagine I told you his wife recently had an upper respiratory tract infection.

Now what is his most likely diagnosis?

An upper respiratory tract infection is most likely.

Imagine now that I told you he has had this cough for 1 year and that he has a 20-pack-year smoking history.

Now what is his most likely diagnosis?

Lung cancer, chronic obstructive pulmonary disease, and/or bronchitis are now more likely.

Each new piece of information increases or decreases the likelihood of a particular scenario within the illness script for cough.

When we can represent something like cough with an illness script, shifting our differential diagnosis or plan as new information is presented becomes much easier. And while we can use our knowledge of pathophysiology to arrive at the same conclusions, illness scripts allow for increased speed, efficiency, and reliability.

Our job as learners is to practice building our library of illness scripts. To do so, we should learn about diseases the same way we want to recall information about them. While we learn, we should practice categorizing information by disease states, with the who, what, when, where, and whys of each disease.

As we build up this library, we need to practice picking up on patterns that will clue us in to what is important and what isn't. And this involves categorizing information as useful or not useful.

Imagine a vignette with ten sentences. You read each sentence with the same amount of energy and attention. But if you could have answered the question after five, does this seem like the most productive use of your time? Would you watch commercials with the same energy and attention as television shows themselves?

When we consider whether information is useful or not, we need to understand why it is, or why it isn't, useful.

What makes a sentence useful?

A useful sentence is one that changes or adds to your working differential. It is a sentence that you need to arrive at or solidify your differential and/or answer choice.

What makes a sentence not useful?

A not useful sentence may be redundant information that does not help you to better solidify your answer choice. Spending time on those sentences that are not useful wastes time and energy.

What makes a sentence a trap?

A trap sentence is any sentence that guides you towards the wrong answer.

How do we know how to identify traps?

If we always knew how to identify the traps, then exams would be easy. But practice should help you to pick up on patterns and increase your likelihood of identifying them.

Now, take a moment to reflect on whether you are the kind of test-taker that incorrectly categorizes information as useful, not useful, or traps. Do you tend to pay attention to aspects of the vignette that steer you towards the wrong answer? Do you fall into traps laid by the test writer? Noticing your own personal patterns will be important to change your approach in the future.

While this may seem laborious, practice will start to shape the way you learn and remember information and will ultimately prove to be worthwhile.

Let's move on to some examples.

Question 1

A 16-year-old girl comes to clinic with her mother due to amenorrhea. She has no medical conditions and takes no medications. She has never been sexually active. Her sister began menstruating at age 13. Temperature is 36.5 °C, blood pressure is 105/60 mmHg, pulse is 55/min, and respirations are 16/min. BMI is 17.5 kg/m². Physical examination reveals few scattered pustules across the face. External genitalia appear normal, but a more detailed pelvic exam is deferred. Tanner stage IV breasts and pubic hair are noted. What is the next best step?

a. Karyotype
b. LH level
c. Pelvic ultrasound
d. Brain MRI
e. Thyroid function studies
f. Detailed dietary history

First, let's prime ourselves by reading the first sentence, the question, and the answer choices. Think of this as an abbreviated version of the 5-Step Approach detailed in Chapter 2.

This reads:

A 16-year-old girl comes to clinic with her mother due to amenorrhea. What is the next best step?

   a. *Karyotype*
   b. *LH level*
   c. *Pelvic ultrasound*
   d. *Brain MRI*
   e. *Thyroid function studies*
   f. *Detailed dietary history*

Let's review the context.

What does the first sentence tell us?

This is an adolescent with amenorrhea. We will need to determine whether this is a primary or secondary amenorrhea.

What do the question and answer choices tell us?

This question wants us to recognize the diagnosis and determine the best test to establish that diagnosis. A question that includes the word "next" will often focus on screening tests and/or stabilization measures and preclude those more advanced imaging techniques or definitive testing.

A detailed dietary history, thyroid function studies, or an LH level are all low risk and noninvasive choices and would thus be reasonable best next steps depending on the scenario. While a karyotype is also a blood test, this is less commonly done, and so we should have a good reason to select this answer.

A brain MRI is the most intensive diagnostic tool of the answer choices. We should only select this answer choice if there is both a good reason to seek out an MRI and there are no other reasonable options for preliminary testing. Imaging, including an MRI or pelvic ultrasound, is more involved than a dietary history or a blood test, and so a screening test, if available, may be a better choice.

Let's try to categorize our answer choices. This will help us to organize the information in the vignette and determine what is useful and what isn't. We can practice breaking up the vignette into more manageable parts.

Can you think of a good way to categorize the answer choices?

Let's form categories based on the type of pathology that can be identified with that diagnostic test.

The categories might read:

   a. Chromosomal abnormality
   b. Anatomic abnormality

    c. Hormonal abnormality specifically related to LH or thyroid
    d. Brain tumor
    e. Abnormality related to diet

Based on these categories, we should be looking for signs of chromosomal, anatomic, hormonal, or dietary abnormalities, or any neurologic signs or symptoms concerning for a brain tumor. Once we establish the diagnosis, we should be able to select an answer choice more easily.

Now we are ready to read through the vignette. Let's read in parts and categorize each part as useful, not useful, or a trap.

She has no medical conditions and takes no medications.

Category: Not useful

Why did the test writer include this?

This sentence would have been more useful if this patient had relevant past medical history or if we were considering a diagnosis that should have presented prior to age 16.

Unless the test writer stated a medical condition that could explain her amenorrhea, or a medical condition that would require medications that could explain her amenorrhea, then this sentence would either be categorized as "not useful" or even "trap." If the test writer had highlighted a specific medical condition, they might be attempting to shift our focus towards a diagnosis that is not actually related to the question as a trap for the test-taker.

There are some medical conditions that might be difficult to recognize as relevant or useful. One example is any autoimmune disorder associated with autoimmune thyroiditis, such as Celiac's disease. If this patient did have a history of Celiac's disease, then this may increase your suspicion for a thyroid abnormality.

She has never been sexually active.

Category: Not useful

Why did the test writer include this?

Pregnancy would be a straightforward reason for this patient's amenorrhea and could be explained by a pelvic ultrasound.

Though we can exclude pregnancy, we cannot exclude ultrasound as an answer choice, as this can be useful to diagnose conditions other than pregnancy.

When pregnancy is suspected, is ultrasound the best next step?

An ultrasound is a non-invasive and gold standard modality to identify and monitor pregnancy. But this is usually not the first test. We will usually obtain a serum or urine pregnancy test first and then confirm an intrauterine pregnancy with an ultrasound.

If we were worried about pregnancy, then pelvic ultrasound would not be the best next step anyway, rendering this information about her sexual history not useful.

Her sister began menstruating at age 13.

Category: Not useful

Why did the test writer include this?

The test writer wants to highlight that this patient might have delayed menarche relative to her sister and thus hint at underlying pathology. However, familial age of menarche is not a reliable tool to determine whether late menarche is pathological. This information does not increase or decrease our suspicion of a particular diagnosis, and therefore is not useful.

If her sister had been 15 years old at the age of menarche, closer to the age of our patient, then this sentence might have been categorized as a "trap," particularly if "reassurance only" was an answer choice.

If her sister had been diagnosed with primary amenorrhea, then we might categorize this sentence as "useful" and explore the possibility of underlying genetic causes.

Temperature is 36.5 °C, blood pressure is 105/60 mmHg, pulse is 55/min, and respirations are 16/min.

Category: Useful

Let's interpret the vitals.

Her temperature is borderline low, her blood pressure is borderline low, and she is bradycardic. Her respiratory rate is normal.

Temperature is rarely low. Most commonly, low temperature is presented in the setting of neonatal sepsis. Adults rarely present with hypothermia. Other reasons for low temperature could include environmental hypothermia, hypothyroidism, or anorexia.

Borderline low blood pressure is non-specific and may be normal. However, we can consider general causes for low blood pressure such as hypovolemia, medications, hormonal abnormalities, or autonomic abnormalities.

The most common population for bradycardia on exams is the elderly due to heart block or a medication side effect. Borderline bradycardia may also be highlighted in athletes. Other reasons might include hypothyroidism and anorexia.

Why did the test writer include these vitals?

These vitals tell the story of a patient with a slowed metabolic rate. These vitals should help narrow our differential and be explained by whatever diagnosis we choose.

| ESHRE/ASRM (Rotterdam) 2003 |
| Two of the three: |
| Clinical and/or biochemical hyperandrogenism (HA) |
| Oligo-/anovulation (OA) |
| Polycystic ovarian morphology (PCOM) |
| **NIH (1990)** |
| To include both: |
| Clinical and/or biochemical hyperandrogenism |
| Oligo-/anovulation |
| **AE-PCOS (2006)** |
| To include both: |
| Clinical and/or biochemical hyperandrogenism |
| Oligo-/anovulation and/or polycystic ovarian morphology |
| **NIH (2012)** |
| To identify one of four phenotypes using Rotterdam criteria |
| HA + OA + PCOM |
| HA + OA |
| HA + PCOM |
| OA + PCOM |

FIGURE 4-2 **Diagnostic Criteria for Polycystic Ovarian Syndrome (PCOS).** (Reproduced with permission from Hoffman BL, Schorge JO, Halvorson LN et al. *Williams Gynecology*, 4th ed. McGraw Hill, 2020.)

BMI is 17.5 kg/m^2.

Category: Useful

Why did the test writer include this?

When the test writer chooses to include BMI, this information will almost always be useful. Usually, this will increase your suspicion about a particular diagnosis.

We already spent some time thinking about possible explanations for her abnormal vital signs, such as hypothyroidism or anorexia. We would expect to see a high BMI in the setting of hypothyroidism and a low BMI in the setting of anorexia. Her vital signs combined with her low BMI are most suggestive of a diagnosis of anorexia. But we should continue to keep an open mind as we read the rest of the vignette.

Physical examination reveals few scattered pustules across the face.

Category: Trap

Why did the test writer include this?

Scattered pustules in the setting of amenorrhea might entice you to consider Polycystic Ovary Syndrome (PCOS) as a possible diagnosis.

The general criteria for PCOS include hyperandrogenism, polycystic ovaries, and amenorrhea or oligomenorrhea (Figure 4-2).

If you were to interpret her acne to represent hyperandrogenism, then we have two answer choices to consider; pelvic ultrasound to evaluate for cystic ovaries (Figure 4-3) or serum LH and FSH testing to evaluate for hyperandrogenism. While we can diagnose hyperandrogenism by appearance alone, serum testing is not an unreasonable consideration if we were worried about PCOS.

When there are two answers that seem equally correct for a particular diagnosis, we can usually generate two conclusions. The first is that the diagnosis is wrong, as it would be impossible to distinguish between the two answer choices. The second is that there is a knowledge gap that would help to select one answer over the other for that diagnosis. We can use other clues in the vignette to tip the scale in one direction or the other.

How suspicious are we of PCOS?

PCOS could not explain her abnormal vital signs and is more often associated with high, rather than low, BMI. While this is not part of the criteria, we should try to identify a diagnosis that explains her low BMI. The diagnosis we choose should be able to explain all, or almost all, of the findings in the vignette. PCOS does not meet these criteria.

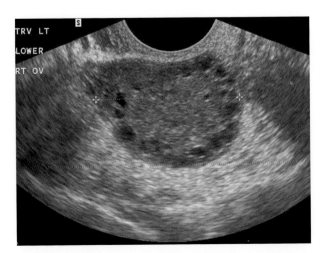

FIGURE 4-3 **Ultrasound Image of a Polycystic Ovary.** (Used with permission from Dr. Elysia Moschos. From Hoffman BL, Schorge JO, Halvorson LN et al. *Williams Gynecology*, 4th ed. McGraw Hill, 2020.)

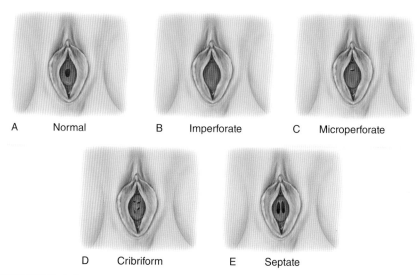

FIGURE 4-4 **Types of Hymen.** A hymen is remnant tissue from embryonic development that normally lines the opening of the vagina. An imperforate hymen is a hymen that covers the entire opening of the vagina and is the most severe type of abnormality. (Reproduced with permission from Hoffman BL, Schorge JO, Halvorson LN et al. *Williams Gynecology*, 4th ed. McGraw Hill, 2020.)

External genitalia appear normal, but a more detailed pelvic exam is deferred.

Category: Trap

Why did the test writer include this?

By telling you that a more detailed pelvic exam was deferred, there remains the possibility that this patient might have an undiagnosed anatomic abnormality like an imperforate hymen (Figure 4-4) or a sex disorder that would require an ultrasound or karyotype. This trap creates doubt for the test-taker.

Tanner stage IV breasts and pubic hair are noted.

Category: Useful

Why did the test writer include this?

If we were considering a chromosomal abnormality such as Turner Syndrome, we might expect delayed or abnormal pubertal development. With normal pubertal development, there is less need for a karyotype.

Now that we've finished the vignette, we can generate a conclusion.

Based on our step-by-step analysis of this vignette, her low BMI and abnormal vital signs suggest that this patient suffers from anorexia, which could also explain her amenorrhea (Figure 4-5).

Anorexia Nervosa (AN)	Bulimia Nervosa (BN)
Physical signs • Significant weight loss unrelated to medical illness • Fat and muscle atrophy • Amenorrhea • Dry hair and skin • Cold, discolored hands and feet • Decreased body temperature • Cold intolerance • Lightheadedness • Decreased ability to concentrate • Bradycardia • Lanugo (fine, baby hair)	**Physical signs** • Swollen parotid glands • Face and extremity edema • Sore throat and chest pain • Fatigue • Bloating, abdominal pain • Diarrhea or constipation • Menstrual irregularities • Callous formation or scars on knuckles (Russell's sign) • Erosion of dental enamel
Behaviors • Severe reduction in food intake • Excessive denial of hunger • Compulsive and/or excessive exercising without signs of fatigue or weakness • Peculiar, ritualistic patterns of food handling • Intense fear of weight gain	**Behaviors** • Exhibits much concern about weight • Eating patterns that alternate between purging and fasting • Depression, guilt, and/or shame especially following a binge

FIGURE 4-5 **Physical Signs and Behaviors of Anorexia and Bulimia Nervosa.** (Reproduced with permission from Hoogenboom BJ, Voight ML, Prentice WE. *Musculoskeletal Interventions: Techniques for Therapeutic Exercise*, 4th ed. McGraw Hill, 2021.)

Why is amenorrhea a feature of anorexia nervosa?

Amenorrhea occurs in anorexia because of the stress on the body, resulting in hypothalamic hypopituitarism. The same phenomenon can be seen in female athletes with a low body weight.

What is the next best step to evaluate for this patient's amenorrhea, if we are most concerned about anorexia?

The best next step would be to ask the patient to complete a food diary. This would help us to better assess whether anorexia nervosa is present. Other possibilities for low weight, such as malabsorptive diseases, may need to be explored in the future if she reports adequate intake.

What is the correct answer?

Detailed dietary history

While there are different variations in how we could have categorized these sentences, the goal is to arrive at the same conclusion. Regardless of how you categorize, you should be using a systematic approach and continue to reassess your differential.

Remember, each sentence should influence the way you interpret and categorize the next. Information is only useful, or not useful, in context, and you need to work to build that context as you read through each vignette.

Question 2

A 25-year-old woman is brought to clinic by her mother for evaluation of her mood. Over the last 2 weeks, her mood has been increasingly anxious. She is convinced that someone has been poisoning their food, and now refuses to eat anything that is not from a sealed package. She has been having difficulty sleeping due to anxiety about this. The patient has never had similar symptoms before. Her past medical history is significant for systemic lupus erythematosus, which was poorly controlled until 3 weeks ago, when she was started on prednisone. Since then, her rash and joint pains have mostly resolved. Vital signs are unremarkable. The patient is agitated and looks around the room frequently. Her mental status exam is otherwise unremarkable. Neurologic exam is grossly normal. What is the most likely diagnosis?

   a. Systemic lupus erythematosus flare
   b. Bipolar I disorder
   c. Bipolar II disorder
   d. Schizophrenia
   e. Medication side effect

First, let's prime ourselves by reading the first sentence and question.

This reads:

A 25-year-old woman is brought to clinic by her mother for evaluation of her mood. What is the most likely diagnosis?

What does the first sentence tell us?

This sentence tells us that her mother is concerned about her mood, though we don't know if the patient herself is concerned. Patients with psychosis often do not recognize their psychotic symptoms as pathologic, which might explain why this adult patient is being brought to clinic by her mother.

What does the question tell us?

We need to determine the diagnosis of this patient.

Now let's read the answer choices. This reads:

   a. *Systemic lupus erythematosus flare*
   b. *Bipolar I disorder*

c. *Bipolar II disorder*
d. *Schizophrenia*
e. *Medication side effect*

What do the answer choices tell us?

There are a few answer choices that are similar to each other while a few stand out. Like the last practice question, we should categorize the answer choices. This will help us more quickly identify the correct answer later.

How would you categorize the answer choices?

The answer choices can be grouped as either a primary psychiatric diagnosis or psychiatric symptom(s) from a medication side effect or medical condition. Establishing these categories is akin to thinking in illness scripts.

Categories with corresponding answer choices are as follows:

a. *Systemic lupus erythematosus flare:* Psychiatric symptom(s) from a medical condition
b. *Bipolar I disorder:* Primary psychiatric diagnosis
c. *Bipolar II disorder:* Primary psychiatric diagnosis
d. *Schizophrenia:* Primary psychiatric diagnosis
e. *Medication side effect:* Psychiatric symptom(s) from a medical condition

Since the majority of the answer choices fall under a primary psychiatric diagnosis, our priority should be to sort information that either supports or doesn't support an answer choice in this category. We can narrow our differential from there.

Notice that both bipolar I and II disorders are both answer choices.

What differentiates bipolar I and II?

The simplest explanation is that bipolar I involves mania, whereas bipolar II involves hypomania and requires the presence of at least one lifetime major depressive episode (Figure 4-6).

Here's how I remember the differences: Bipolar I is more severe and thus includes mania. It is number 1, representing the first most severe of the two. Because of the severity of mania, depression is not a requirement. But because bipolar II only involves hypomania, depression must be present. Bipolar II represents the second most severe of the two.

Is schizophrenia similar to bipolar disorder?

Both bipolar I disorder and schizophrenia can involve psychotic and depressive features. The psychotic features can be quite similar, but the depressive features are more distinct.

Bipolar I Disorder	1 or more manic or mixed episodes, usually accompanied by major depressive episode *Subtypes:* Mixed Episode, Rapid Cycling
Bipolar II Disorder	1 or more major depressive episodes accompanied by at least 1 hypomanic episode
Cyclothymic Disorder	At least 2y of chronic fluctuations between dysthymic & hypomanic symptoms Symptoms do not meet criteria for mania or major depressive episode
Bipolar Disorder NOS	Symptoms do not meet the criteria for any specific bipolar disorder

FIGURE 4-6 **Comparing Bipolar Disorder Types.** The key difference between bipolar disorders is the presence of mania in bipolar I. When only hypomania is present, major depressive episodes must also be present to establish a diagnosis of bipolar II. (Reproduced with permission from Attridge RL, Miller ML, Moote R, Ryan L. *Internal Medicine: A Guide to Clinical Therapeutics.* McGraw Hill, 2013.)

The depressive features in schizophrenia are classified more so as "negative symptoms," whereas the depression we see in bipolar disorder should fulfill the SIG E CAPS criteria (Sleep, Interest, Guilt, Energy, Concentration, Appetite, Psychomotor, Suicidality). The negative symptoms of schizophrenia must be present to establish a diagnosis, whereas depression does not need to be present in bipolar I disorder.

What are negative symptoms?

Negative symptoms are just as they sound: The absence of something; absence of pleasure in doing things, absence of speech, absence of social interaction, etc. (Figure 4-7).

There are also differences in terms of the length of time needed to make a diagnosis based on *DSM-5* criteria, but these are always hard to recall.

Can you remember the duration of symptoms needed for a diagnosis of depression, bipolar disorder, and schizophrenia?

Depression can be diagnosed after only 2 weeks and bipolar disorder after only 1 week of mania. But schizophrenia requires 6 months for a diagnosis.

- Disorganized thinking and speech, with fragmented logic, frequent derailment, or incoherence
- Auditory hallucinations that make little or no sense
- Grossly disorganized or catatonic behavior
- Fragmented delusions that are illogical
- Affect flattening, alogia, or avolition

FIGURE 4-7 *DSM-5* **Criteria for Schizophrenia.** (Reproduced with permission from Brust JCM. *CURRENT Diagnosis & Treatment: Neurology,* 3rd ed. McGraw Hill, 2019; and data from American Psychiatric Association. *Diagnostic and Statistical Manual of Mental Disorders,* 5th ed. American Psychiatric Association Publishing, 2013.)

What about the answer choices that do not fall under the primary psychiatric diagnosis category?

We should pay attention to any medical conditions she has and medications that she is taking, with special attention to the temporal association of medications and her symptoms. The challenge will be to determine whether this information is useful, not useful, or a trap.

Now we are ready to read through the vignette. Again, let's identify sentences as "Useful, Not Useful, or Trap."

Over the last 2 weeks, her mood has been increasingly anxious.

Category: Useful.

Why did the test writer include this?

This sentence provides us with the timeline.

How does this timeline narrow our differential?

We know that schizophrenia requires a longer timeframe to make a diagnosis, so we can eliminate this diagnosis as an option. However, bipolar disorders I and II remain possible choices given the 2-week timeframe.

Does the presence of anxiety help to narrow our differential?

Not really. Based on our preparation, we know that the presence or absence of anxiety is not useful to us. This is an example of a sentence that may have seemed useful had we not done the preparation ahead of time.

Why did the test writer include this?

Any piece of information that is not useful but not a trap, like the mention of her anxiety, is included to challenge your ability to sift through and correctly categorize information as important or unimportant. The ability to do so is an important test-taking skill.

She is convinced that someone has been poisoning their food, and now refuses to eat anything that is not from a sealed package.

Category: Useful

Why did the test writer include this?

This sentence provides us with key information to characterize her mood disturbance. These thoughts can be categorized as delusional, and delusions fall under the category of psychosis.

How does this change our differential?

The presence of psychotic features eliminates bipolar II disorder as a likely option. Now that we are no longer considering bipolar II disorder, we no longer need to look for signs of depression.

Out of the "primary psychiatric diagnosis" category, only bipolar I disorder remains.

She has been having difficulty sleeping due to anxiety about this.

Category: Trap

Why did the test writer include this?

If we were still considering bipolar II as a potential answer, then we might start to think that this difficulty sleeping represents a feature of depression. However, we should remember that depression can be concurrently present in many disorders, including bipolar I disorder. Sleeplessness can also be a feature of mania, not just depression. We must be careful not to anchor on any particular diagnosis from this information and fall into test writer traps. Once we start anchoring on an incorrect diagnosis, it becomes harder to reverse our thought processes. Anchoring will be discussed in more detail in Chapter 5.

The patient has never had similar symptoms before.

Category: Not useful

Why did the test writer include this?

While this information might be important to note, it will not alter our differential and is therefore not useful.

Her past medical history is significant for systemic lupus erythematosus, which was poorly controlled until 3 weeks ago, when she was started on prednisone.

Category: Useful

This sentence is rich with information. Let's break it up into three parts.

Her past medical history is significant for systemic lupus erythematosus…

Why did the test writer include this?

Based on the answer choices, we knew that this patient would have a past medical history of something that might be able to explain her symptoms.

If you recall, lupus can cause mood changes. But this also could very easily be a trap by the test writer.

… which was poorly controlled until 3 weeks ago…

Why did the test writer include this?

We should always pay attention whenever test writers refer to time. In this case, the test writer is telling us that a change occurred 3 weeks ago. This is around the time her symptoms began.

Does this support or contradict the idea that lupus is the cause of her mood disturbance?

If we pay close attention to this part of the sentence, the test writer is saying that her lupus has been better controlled over the last 3 weeks. It therefore would seem unlikely that she has developed a lupus-associated mood disturbance and/or psychosis in the setting of symptom improvement. In fact, based on the time-line alone, we should eliminate this as a possibility.

…when she was started on prednisone.

Why did the test writer include this?

Well, we now know that this patient was started on a new medication 3 weeks ago. Any time a new medication is started, we should consider whether this could explain the patient's presentation.

On medical board exams, if the timeline matches, then there is a high probability that the two are related. However, there is always the remote possibility that this is a trap.

We should always use a combination of medical knowledge and probabilities to make the best choices on exam day.

In this case, we should consider whether prednisone is associated with mood disturbances.

Spoiler alert: Prednisone can cause psychosis.

But what if you didn't know that prednisone can cause psychosis?

When there is no other answer choice that fits well, medication side effect is often a good guess, particularly in this case. While I am not usually in support of the process of elimination, there are some instances where it is useful.

Let's continue with the vignette.

Since then, her rash and joint pains have mostly resolved.

Category: Not useful

Why did the test writer include this?

Much of vignettes are redundant. In this case, we already know from the last sentence that her lupus is better controlled.

Vital signs are unremarkable.

Category: Not useful

None of the diagnoses we are considering would require vital sign abnormalities.

The patient is agitated and looks around the room frequently.

Category: Not useful

Why did the test writer include this?

While a stretch, if someone was considering bipolar II as a possible answer choice, then this patient's psychomotor agitation could fulfill one of the SIG E CAPS criteria for depression. But for those who are no longer considering depression and bipolar II disorder, then this sentence is just another time- and energy-waster.

Her mental status exam is otherwise unremarkable. Neurologic exam is grossly normal.

Category: Useful

Why did the test writer include this?

For a patient with schizophrenia or mania, we might expect more pronounced exam findings. In terms of schizophrenia, we should expect some "negative symptoms" as discussed earlier. And for bipolar I disorder, we might expect racing thoughts or behaviors.

Now that we have finished reading the vignette, we are ready to select our answer choice. Let's remind ourselves of the original categories we came up with. These included a primary psychiatric diagnosis or psychiatric symptom(s) from a medication side effect or medical condition.

There is not enough support in the vignette to establish any primary psychiatric diagnosis except for possibly delusional disorder, but this is not an answer choice. Remember, the test writer should always give adequate support for the correct answer choice.

Additionally, recall that one of the key features of psychiatric diagnoses is that the symptoms are not better explained or caused by a medication or medical condition. It would seem highly coincidental for a new psychiatric disorder to start 1 week after starting a new medication. And we discussed that her symptoms are very unlikely to be attributed to her lupus, as the test writer highlights the improvement in her lupus symptoms.

Based on our reasoning, there is a high probability of a medication side effect causing her psychosis; in this case, prednisone. And psychosis is, indeed, a side effect of prednisone.

What is the correct answer?

Medication side effect

For this question, the challenge was picking out the few important details that were needed to answer this question correctly. These details could have easily been missed. On the flip side, this question could have been answered with only a few of the details found in the vignette. It was important to prepare prior to reading the vignette so that we were able to easily pick out those details.

Question 3

A 24-year-old man presents to the emergency room due to a cat bite on his left hand. His cat attacked him at home after he picked up his cat's food bowl while she was still eating. His hand initially became swollen and red. It became progressively difficult for him to move his middle and index fingers. He presented to the emergency room today due to severe pain and inability to use the hand. Temperature is 38°C, blood pressure is 120/80 mmHg, pulse is 75/min, respirations are 16/min. On exam, there are two linear lacerations overlying the dorsal aspect of his 2nd and 3rd metacarpal joints. There is marked surrounding swelling and erythema. There is pain with passive motion of his 2nd and 3rd fingers. Which of the following is the best next step in management?

a. Oral antibiotic therapy and outpatient follow-up
b. Surgical irrigation and debridement
c. Repair the laceration
d. Immunization for rabies
e. Supportive care only

For this example, we should practice identifying the important information and why pieces of information are, or aren't, important. Our focus should be on how new information is going to change our differential and/or our management plan. To do this, we can evaluate whether that information supports or contradicts each answer choice.

What are the most important features from the vignette?

The most important features from the vignette might include:

1. 24-year-old man
2. Provoked cat bite on left hand
3. Lacerations over the 2nd and 3rd metacarpal joints
4. Swelling, redness, severe pain, and limited range of motion
5. Febrile with otherwise normal vital signs

How would you summarize this scenario?

A 24-year-old man presents after a provoked cat bite, with exam notable for fever, lacerations, swelling, redness, and severe pain with limited range of motion of the 2nd and 3rd metacarpal joints.

Now let's review the answer choices.

As a reminder, the answer choices read:

a. *Oral antibiotic therapy and outpatient follow-up*
b. *Surgical irrigation and debridement*
c. *Repair the laceration*

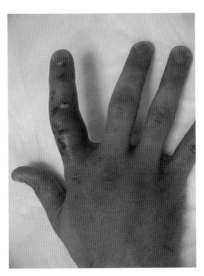

FIGURE 4-8 **Infected Finger From an Animal Bite.** Notice the increased redness, significant swelling, and pus at one of the puncture sites. (Reproduced with permission from Sherman SC. *Simon's Emergency Orthopedics*, 8th ed. McGraw Hill, 2019.)

    d. *Immunization for rabies*
    e. *Supportive care only*

Notice how the answer choices do not include diagnoses but rather management approaches.

If we want to assign points to each answer choice, we first need to identify the condition(s) that each answer choice refers to.

Can you assign possible diagnoses to each answer choice?

This might look something like this:

    a. *Oral antibiotic therapy and outpatient follow-up*: Mild to moderate bacterial wound infection (Figure 4-8)
    b. *Surgical irrigation and debridement*: Moderate to severe bacterial infection that may include drug-resistant bacteria and/or joint involvement
    c. *Repair the laceration*: Focus on a large wound/laceration rather than an infection
    d. *Immunization for rabies*: Biggest concern is for rabies
    e. *Supportive care only*: Small wound not requiring irritation or suturing and no concern for infection (Figure 4-9).

From the answer choices, we have generated a few differential diagnoses:

    1. Mild to moderate bacterial wound infection
    2. Drug-resistant bacterial wound infection

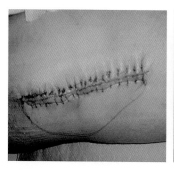 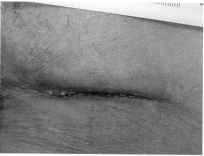

FIGURE 4-9 **Uninfected Wound(s).** Notice how there is no significant erythema with only mild discoloration surrounding the wound, consistent with normal healing. (Reproduced with permission from Hamm RL. *Text and Atlas of Wound Diagnosis and Treatment*, 2nd ed. McGraw Hill, 2019.)

3. Septic joint
4. Large laceration
5. Rabies risk
6. Small, uninfected wound

We should take a moment to note the key features of each diagnosis. This will allow us to easily match new information to a respective diagnosis and add up points for or against a diagnosis, and by extension, an answer choice.

This might look something like this:

1. Bacterial wound infection: When considering a bacterial wound infection, we should differentiate between inflammation and infection. Inflammation can cause redness, swelling, itching, discomfort, and pain, but these are all typically mild. Excessive redness, purulence, drainage, and abscess formation are more suggestive of a bacterial infection, as is the presence of a fever. An animal bite is rich with bacteria and increases the probability that a bacterial wound infection will develop.
2. Drug-resistant bacterial wound infection: A drug-resistant infection can be identified from a culture. However, we can also diagnose this clinically if a patient fails antibiotics, though sometimes there is treatment failure because of the presence of an abscess that requires drainage due to inadequate antibiotic penetration.
3. Septic joint: Consider how an infected joint would present. If there is increased swelling and fluid in the joint, then we would expect limited and painful range of motion. If only the soft tissue surrounding the joint is infected, then we would not expect symptoms to be significantly worsened with movement.
4. Large laceration: A large laceration should be repaired in many cases but is often avoided in the case of an animal bite. This is because of the introduction of bacteria from the animal. Wound closure seals in bacteria and

increases the risk of treatment failure. However, there are some exceptions, such as facial wounds, for cosmesis.

5. Rabies risk: Classically, we worry about rabies when there is a bat, racoon, or squirrel, but should always be considered with cats and dogs. With any animal bite, the key question is whether this was a provoked or unprovoked attack. An unprovoked attack is more concerning for rabies. While a provoked animal bite can still be from a rabid animal, there would be less of a concern.

6. Small, uninfected wound: Normal signs of inflammation, such as mild redness, swelling, itching, discomfort, and pain would suggest an uninfected wound. If small, this would not require any kind of repair.

Now let's match each diagnosis with features from the vignette that support or contradict a given diagnosis. For example, the presence of severe pain might support the diagnosis of a bacterial wound infection but contradict the presence of an uninfected wound. After we complete this exercise, we can determine which diagnosis has the most support.

1. Bacterial wound infection
   (+) Severe pain
   (+) Swollen, red
   (+) Cat bite
   (+) Fever

2. Drug-resistant bacterial wound infection
   (−) No prior antibiotic trial
   (−) No culture

3. Septic joint
   (+) Swollen, red
   (+) Limited range of motion
   (+) Severe pain
   (+) Cat bite
   (+) Fever
   (+) Location of the wound over the joint

4. Large laceration
   (−) No mention of hemostasis problems
   (−) No mention of laceration length or depth

5. Rabies risk
   (−) Unprovoked bite

6. Small, uninfected wound
   (+) Swollen, red
   (−) Severe pain
   (−) Limited range of motion
   (−) Presence of fever

When we do this exercise, the correct answer choice should have the most supporting evidence and very little evidence that contradicts that answer choice. Even if your own fund of knowledge is lacking, the hope is that enough points will still lead you to the correct answer.

If there is no clear correct answer, then it is likely you either misunderstood the vignette or have a poor grasp of one of the answer choices. This should prompt you to reevaluate your reasoning to see if you end up with a different result.

Based on this strategy for this vignette, we can see that the best supported diagnoses are bacterial wound infection or septic joint.

A bacterial wound infection is likely present. But is there also a septic joint?

What is a key difference between the presentation of a wound infection and a joint infection?

The most important difference is the presence of pain with passive range of motion and/or reduced mobility, because this would indicate that the joint is involved.

The test writer made a point to note the location of the wound over the joint as well as symptoms suggesting joint involvement. This is enough to support a septic joint.

Now that we feel confident with our diagnosis, let's answer the question. As a reminder, the answer choices read:

a. *Oral antibiotic therapy and outpatient follow-up*
b. *Surgical irrigation and debridement*
c. *Repair the laceration*
d. *Immunization for rabies*
e. *Supportive care only*

While appropriate for a wound infection, oral antibiotic therapy and outpatient follow-up are not sufficient treatment for a septic joint. We need to escalate treatment given the joint involvement.

What is the correct answer?

Surgical irrigation and debridement

When you are stuck, you can always rely on this approach to provide a more quantitative measure for the most likely answer choice.

Question 4

A 43-year-old female is seen in the emergency room for fever. She has felt feverish since yesterday. She became concerned this morning when she measured a temperature of 102 °F and decided to come to the emergency room. She was recently diagnosed with Stage IV ovarian cancer and her last session of chemotherapy was 1 week ago. She underwent tumor debulking 4 weeks ago for symptom management and had been recovering well from the surgery until yesterday. The patient also has a history of asthma and takes an inhaled gluco-corticoid daily and a bronchodilator as needed. Temperature is 101.9 °F, blood pressure is 105/80 mmHg, and pulse is 100/min. She is thin appearing on exam. White patches are noted on the oral mucosa and tongue. Her peripherally inserted central venous catheter site is mildly erythematous without discharge or tenderness to palpation. Abdominal exam is notable for palpable masses in the left lower abdomen with mild tenderness. Surgical incision overlying the abdomen is well healed with minimal erythema and no drainage. Pelvic exam demonstrates no vulvar erythema or cervical motion tenderness. Initial blood culture results show *Candida* growth. Which of the following is the most likely source of the blood culture results?

a. Oropharyngeal infection
b. Vulvovaginitis
c. Contaminated sample
d. Central venous catheter
e. Post-operative infection

Again, let's practice identifying key information in the vignette and assigning points that support or contradict each answer choice.

What are the key features from the vignette?

The most important features from the vignette might include:

1. 43-year-old female
2. Ovarian cancer
3. Last chemotherapy 1 week ago
4. Tumor debulking 4 weeks ago
5. History of asthma on daily steroid and bronchodilator as needed
6. Vital signs concerning for sepsis
7. Oral white patches
8. Mild erythema surrounding central venous catheter
9. Abdominal masses and tenderness
10. Well-healed surgical incision with minimal erythema
11. Normal pelvic exam
12. *Candida* positive blood culture

This vignette presents an added challenge because of the complicated timeline.

How would we summarize the timeline?

This patient underwent tumor debulking 4 weeks ago. Her last chemotherapy session was 1 week ago. She was feeling well until yesterday, when she developed a fever.

We should also characterize each answer choice with a few facts about each.

As a reminder, the answer choices read:

a. *Oropharyngeal infection*
b. *Vulvovaginitis*
c. *Contaminated sample*
d. *Central venous catheter*
e. *Post-operative infection*

This might look something like this:

a. *Oropharyngeal infection:* In the case of this vignette, the test writer is likely referring to the white patches described on her oral mucosa. Based on the description, the test writer seems to be alluding to oropharyngeal candidiasis, or oral thrush (Figure 4-10). Immunocompromised patients are at higher risk of developing thrush.
b. *Vulvovaginitis:* We might expect increased vaginal discharge, possibly a foul odor, pain, itching, and/or visible redness on exam (Figure 4-11).
c. *Contaminated sample:* The most common way a test writer will test your ability to distinguish between a true bacteremia or fungemia and a contaminated sample will be based on the clinical appearance of the patient and the type of organism. *Staph epidermidis* is the most tested contaminant.
d. *Central venous catheter:* This should always be a consideration in any patient with a fever and a central line. Local signs of infection may or may not be present around the catheter.
e. *Post-operative infection:* We would expect significant tenderness around the incision with marked redness and sometimes drainage or fluctuance (Figure 4-12). We would also expect this type of infection to become symptomatic 1 to 2 weeks following surgery.

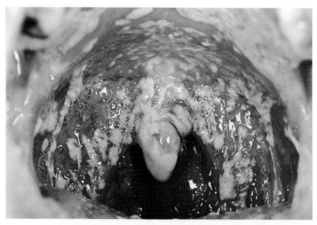

FIGURE 4-10 **Oral Candidiasis.** White patches can be seen throughout the oral mucosa. (Used with permission from Lawrence B. Stack, MD. From Knoop KJ, Stack LB, Storrow AB, Thurman RJ. *The Atlas of Emergency Medicine*, 5th ed. McGraw Hill, 2021.)

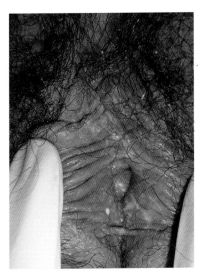

FIGURE 4-11 **Vulvovaginal Candidiasis.** White patches with erythema can be seen on the vulva and introitus. (Used with permission from Richard P. Usatine, MD. From Usatine RP, Smith MA, Mayeaux EJ, Jr, Chumley HS. *The Color Atlas & Synopsis of Family Medicine*, 3rd ed. McGraw Hill, 2019.)

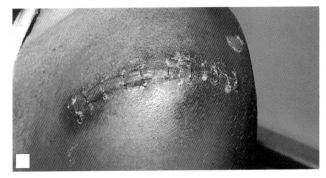

FIGURE 4-12 **Infected Wound.** Notice how there is significant erythema extending from the incision with surrounding swelling, concerning for infection. Inflammation associated with normal healing should be minimal with only mild swelling and erythema. (Used with permission from Matthew D. Sztajnkrycer, MD, PhD. From Knoop KJ, Stack LB, Storrow AB, Thurman RJ. *The Atlas of Emergency Medicine*, 5th ed. McGraw Hill, 2021.)

We can combine the first two steps by listing the key facts we pulled from the vignette under each answer choice to evaluate what diagnosis is best supported.

This would look something like this:

  a. *Oropharyngeal infection*
    (+) Immunosuppression
    (+) Daily inhaled steroid

   (+) Oral white patches
   (−) Vital signs concerning for sepsis
   (−) Presence of fungemia

b. *Vulvovaginitis*
   (+) Immunosuppression
   (−) Vital signs concerning for sepsis
   (−) Normal pelvic exam
   (−) Presence of fungemia

c. *Contaminated sample*
   (+) Organism type
   (−) Vital signs concerning for sepsis

d. *Central venous catheter*
   (+) Immunosuppression
   (+) Vital signs concerning for sepsis
   (+) Organism type
   (+/−) Mild surrounding erythema

e. *Post-operative infection*
   (+) Vital signs concerning for sepsis
   (+) Abdominal tenderness near incision site
   (−) Minimal redness
   (−) No drainage
   (−) Well healed incision
   (−) 4 weeks after surgery

If we review the evidence in this case, this patient's central venous catheter appears to be the most likely source of her *Candida* blood stream infection, followed in close second by oropharyngeal infection.

Let's reason through the two best supported options to arrive at the correct answer.

Consider an oropharyngeal infection. As mentioned earlier, white patches are classic for a *Candida* infection. Risk factors include an immunocompromised state or the use of inhaled corticosteroids. The patient in this vignette has both risk factors. All signs suggest that this patient does indeed have an oropharyngeal infection.

However, we should remind ourselves of the question. The question asks for the most likely source of the blood culture results. While an oropharyngeal infection may very well be present, this is not the likely cause of her candidemia. More likely, her oral thrush is a trap set by the test writer.

Now consider a central venous catheter infection. We know that a central line increases the risk of a blood stream infection. Her immunocompromised state increases her risk of infection even more, especially for less common infections like *Candida*.

Is there any other support for her central venous catheter causing her blood stream infection?

The vignette mentions some mild erythema around the central line. While this could be related to her fungemia, it could represent mild irritation from the line. We don't know if this is useful, not useful, or a trap. Regardless, we know that you do not need skin erythema surrounding a line to diagnose a central line infection, and therefore do not need this information to answer the question.

What is the correct answer?

Central venous catheter

There are many ways to tackle a vignette. We used a combination of reasoning and listing out important features from the vignette that support or contradict the answer choices. As you practice your test-taking skills, you will become more comfortable combining approaches. Keep in mind that there will always be more than one way to answer a question. The best approach is what works best for you and for the question in front of you.

Question 5

A 35-year-old female comes to the emergency department due to severe right lower quadrant pain. She has noticed intermittent right lower abdominal pain over the past few days. However, her pain became constant and severe this morning while on her daily jog. She has had multiple episodes of emesis on her way to the emergency department. The patient is sexually active and has been trying to conceive with her husband. She has been undergoing fertility treatments for the last 3 months. She cannot remember her last period. Temperature 37 °C, blood pressure 100/70 mmHg, pulse is 100/min. She is ill-appearing. There is exquisite tenderness to palpation and a palpable mass in the right lower quadrant. There is no guarding or rebound. She is morbidly obese. Urine pregnancy test is negative. Which of the following additional information would be most helpful in establishing this patient's diagnosis?

a. Past medical history
b. Number of sexual partners
c. Urinary symptoms
d. Past surgical history
e. Family history of malignancy

Again, let's practice identifying key information in the vignette and assigning points that support or contradict each answer choice.

Recall the first step is to list the main features of this vignette.

What are the who, what, when, where, and whys of this vignette?

Who: 35-year-old female

What: Localized abdominal pain, was intermittent, now severe, provoked by activity, emesis present, no rebound or guarding

When: Acute

Where: Emergency room and right lower quadrant

Why: What is the patient's diagnosis?

The next step is to review and characterize each answer choice. We should try to determine what diagnoses are being referenced by each answer choice.

Let's review the answer choices and work through this problem:

a. *Past medical history:* We won't be able to consider this answer choice further until we read the vignette.
b. *Number of sexual partners:* Knowing the number of sexual partners could be useful if we suspect a sexually transmitted infection.
c. *Urinary symptoms:* The presence of urinary symptoms would be important if we suspected a urinary tract infection.
d. *Past surgical history:* Like past medical history, we won't be able to consider this answer choice further until we read the vignette. We can keep in mind that the most commonly tested risk factor for small bowel obstruction is history of prior abdominal surgery.
e. *Family history of malignancy:* This is important if we suspect malignancy, especially those cancers that tend to have a genetic association, such as colon, ovarian, or breast cancer.

These answer choices were not especially helpful in preparing us for the vignette but will hopefully be useful later to narrow in on a diagnosis. Because the answer choices weren't very useful, we will have to focus on key information from the vignette.

Now we are ready to read the vignette and identify important features.

When we are reviewing the vignette, we can think in terms of "pertinent positives" and "pertinent negatives." A "pertinent positive" is a finding that is present, whereas a "pertinent negative" is when a finding is absent, and the presence or absence of those findings is important in determining your diagnosis.

What are some pertinent positives from the vignette?

Pertinent positives:

1. Unknown last menstrual period
2. Morbidly obese with oligomenorrhea and infertility
3. Undergoing fertility treatment
4. Localized pain to the right lower quadrant
5. Exquisite tenderness to palpation

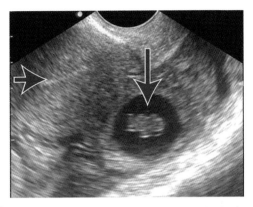

FIGURE 4-13 **Ultrasound Image of Ectopic Pregnancy.** The horizontal arrow points towards an empty uterus. Note the thin endometrial stripe. The vertical arrow points towards an embryo in the adnexa. (Adapted with permission from Ma OJ, Mateer JR, Reardon RF et al. *Ma and Mateer's Emergency Ultrasound*, 3rd ed. McGraw Hill, 2014.)

6. Palpable mass
7. Hypotensive and tachycardic

What are some pertinent negatives from the vignette?

Pertinent negatives:

1. Afebrile
2. Urine pregnancy test negative
3. No guarding or rebound

Let's assign some possible diagnoses to each pertinent positive and negative. We will then be able to look for patterns and later return to our list of answer choices.

Pertinent positives:

1. Unknown last menstrual period: Ectopic pregnancy (Figure 4-13), uterine pregnancy, or oligomenorrhea
2. Morbidly obese with oligomenorrhea and infertility: Polycystic ovarian syndrome
3. Fertility treatments: Risk of ectopic pregnancy or ovarian cysts or uterine pregnancy
4. Localized pain: Appendicitis, ruptured cyst, ectopic pregnancy, malignancy, pelvic inflammatory disease, tubo-ovarian abscess, ovarian torsion, or nephrolithiasis
5. Exquisite tenderness to palpation: Possible surgical abdomen, high acuity
6. Palpable mass: Malignancy, cyst, ectopic pregnancy, uterine pregnancy, large stool burden, or tubo-ovarian abscess
7. Mildly hypotensive and tachycardic: Dehydration, hemorrhage, sepsis (Figure 4-14), or pregnancy

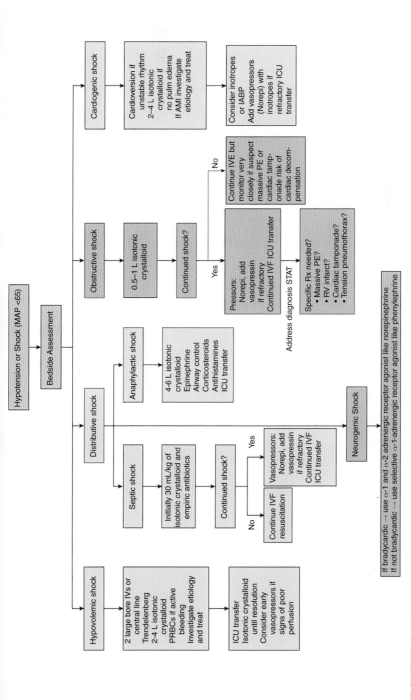

FIGURE 4-14 Management of Types of Shock. The four categories for shock include hypovolemic, distributive, obstructive, and cardiogenic. Distributive shock refers to shock caused by vasodilation and is broken down further into septic and anaphylactic shock. Obstructive shock refers to shock caused by physical obstruction to blood flow at the level of the great vessels or heart itself. Examples include tension pneumothorax, pulmonary embolism, and cardiac tamponade. (Reproduced with permission from McKean SC, Ross JJ, Dressler DD, Scheurer DB. *Principles and Practice of Hospital Medicine*, 2nd ed. McGraw Hill, 2017.)

Pertinent negatives:

1. Afebrile: Unlikely infectious
2. No guarding or rebound: Appendicitis or peritonitis unlikely
3. Urine pregnancy test negative: Pregnancy unlikely

What are the diagnoses we generated?

The possible diagnoses we identified include: ectopic pregnancy, uterine pregnancy, malignancy, cyst, polycystic ovary syndrome, appendicitis, nephrolithiasis, pelvic inflammatory disease, tubo-ovarian abscess, ovarian torsion, and constipation.

What diagnoses are ruled out by the "pertinent negatives" that we identified?

An infectious or inflammatory process such as tubo-ovarian abscess, pelvic inflammatory disease, or appendicitis is unlikely, as is pregnancy.

And while actually a "pertinent positive," the high acuity of her presentation suggests against constipation.

If we exclude those diagnoses, we are left with malignancy, cyst, polycystic ovary syndrome, nephrolithiasis, and ovarian torsion.

Now that we have a list of possible diagnoses, we are finally ready to list those features from the vignette that support or contradict a given diagnosis.

1. *Malignancy*
    (+) Palpable mass
    (−) Acuity
    (−) No "red flag" symptoms (weight loss, early satiety)
    (−) Age

2. *Ovarian torsion*
    (+) Age
    (+) Acuity
    (+) Onset with or worsened by activity
    (+) Emesis
    (+) Higher risk of ovarian cysts
    (+) Location of pain
    (+) Palpable mass

3. *Ruptured ovarian cyst*
    (+) Age
    (+) Acuity
    (+) Onset with or worsened by activity
    (+) Emesis
    (+) Higher risk of ovarian cysts
    (+) Location of pain

   (−) No peritoneal signs
   (−) Pain seems out of proportion

4. *Nephrolithiasis*
   (+) Acuity
   (+) Pain
   (−) Lack of genitourinary symptoms
   (−) Palpable mass
   (−) Ill appearing

5. *Polycystic ovary syndrome*
   (+) Oligomenorrhea
   (+) Infertility
   (+) Obesity
   (−) Age

The most well-supported diagnoses are polycystic ovary syndrome, ovarian torsion, and ruptured ovarian cyst.

Let's think through these diagnoses individually.

Is her polycystic ovary syndrome related to her acute presentation?

It seems unlikely that polycystic ovary syndrome itself is causing her acute symptoms directly.

We know from the name alone that someone with polycystic ovary syndrome is more likely to have, well, many cysts on their ovaries. The fact that she is undergoing infertility treatment also predisposes her to ovarian cysts. If we know she is at risk of having cystic ovaries, then it would not be unreasonable to suspect that one of them ruptured.

Is she at risk of ovarian torsion?

Yes! Imagine you hang a small ball from the ceiling with a string and there is a strong gust of wind. The small ball and string will move easily and together in the direction of the wind. Now imagine the ball is much larger and wind blows on the string. The string will likely move in the direction of the wind, but the heavy ball is more likely to pull in a different direction, increasing the risk that the ball twists around the string. The same phenomenon can occur with ovarian cysts, which is why cysts are a risk factor for ovarian torsion.

Now that we have narrowed our differential diagnoses to ovarian torsion and ruptured ovarian cyst, let's review the answer choices again.

a. *Past medical history*: We established that this patient's polycystic ovary syndrome and infertility treatments predispose her to ovarian cysts and ovarian torsion. This answer seems likely.

b. *Number of sexual partners*: As we are not suspicious of sexually transmitted infections, pelvic inflammatory disease, or tubo-ovarian abscess, her sexual history is not relevant.

c. *Genitourinary symptoms*: We are not suspicious of urinary tract infection or nephrolithiasis.

d. *Past surgical history:* We are not concerned about any diagnoses that might result from prior surgical history, such as a small bowel obstruction.

e. *Family history:* We are not as concerned about malignancy. While we could argue for this possibility, there is far more support for ovarian torsion or ovarian cyst, and we should focus on the best supported answer.

What is the correct answer?

Past medical history

Because of the way we broke down the vignette and answer choices, it was easy to identify the most important information. And while it may seem that you won't have time to go through this process on exam day, enough practice will build up your library of illness scripts and allow this process to occur automatically.

SUMMARY

1. Understanding context is the first step to identifying important information.
2. Illness scripts represent our knowledge about a disease as an organized summary.
3. Illness scripts allow for increased speed, efficiency, and reliability.
4. Practice breaking up information into manageable parts, like the who, what, when, where, and whys of each disease.
5. When in doubt, the best way to identify something as useful, not useful, or a trap is to consider why the test writer chose to include that information.
6. Each sentence should influence the way you interpret and categorize the next.

5

Anchoring

INTRODUCTION

Anchoring is a term you start to hear a lot more as you begin your clinical rotations.

Attendings will advise you to avoid anchoring on a diagnosis. I call this the "bad" kind of anchoring.

The "bad" kind of anchoring is a bias that occurs when we anchor on a particular reference point or conclusion. After we "anchor," subsequent information is interpreted or understood differently based on this bias. When we anchor on a diagnosis prematurely, we are at risk of ignoring or misinterpreting contradictory information.

The propensity to anchor is described as a test-taking weakness:

> *"Learners who exhibit this deficiency make an early decision on the diagnosis, ignore or downplay information inconsistent with the diagnosis, and may list facts that are inconsistent with the chosen diagnosis or simply fail to note the inconsistencies."*[1]

You may recall earlier advice detailed throughout this book, especially in Chapter 2, to "anchor" on a diagnosis or conclusion. This is the "good" kind of anchoring. This advice is designed to prevent new information from confusing you or clouding your judgment after having made a conclusion.

What is the difference between the "good" and the "bad" kind of anchoring?

The "good" kind of anchoring should provide you with enough confidence in your conclusion, but not so much that you ignore new, pertinent information. We want to remain flexible enough to carefully consider whether new information should affect our conclusions.

We need to learn to strike a balance between the "good" and the "bad" kind of anchoring.

Let's work through an example.

Imagine a female patient presents to the emergency department with right lower abdominal pain for one day. It is severe and sharp. The pain was more diffuse earlier in the day and now feels more localized to the right lower quadrant. She has had a loss of appetite and one episode of emesis just prior to her arrival in the emergency department.

Do you know what the diagnosis might be?

Most of us probably suspect appendicitis. This is a common diagnosis and everything we know so far fits.

The "good" kind of anchoring will help us to focus our attention and stay on track. But the "bad" kind of anchoring could bias us towards appendicitis before we have enough information to make a conclusion.

We don't know yet if the correct diagnosis is indeed appendicitis.

What are some other possible diagnoses?

This patient might have ovarian torsion, a tubo-ovarian abscess, malignancy, or even just severe constipation.

Imagine we learn that the patient is afebrile and tachycardic.

How do her vital signs change your differential?

Appendicitis often presents with fever, though not always. This information decreases the likelihood of appendicitis. But the "bad" kind of anchoring might influence us to continue to focus on a diagnosis of appendicitis despite the absence of a fever.

The "bad" kind of anchoring makes us less flexible in response to new information that should change our differential.

"Good" anchoring has a similar purpose: To make it harder to change our minds in light of new information. But "good" anchoring occurs after we have gathered enough evidence to support our conclusion(s) and should always be flexible enough to be changed in light of new and convincing information.

We need to hone our test-taking skills to avoid "bad" anchoring and instead use "good" anchoring to our advantage.

All of us will "bad" anchor many times in our medical careers. The most important thing is that we recognize when this happens and try to prevent this bias in the future.

Let's go through a few board-style practice questions.

Question 1

A 17-year-old girl is brought to clinic by her mother for increased thirst and lethargy. Over the last two days, she has become increasingly thirsty and has been urinating more frequently. The mother is concerned that she has a urinary tract infection. Her past medical history is notable for hypothyroidism and fibromyalgia. Temperature is 37 °C, blood pressure is 95/70 mmHg, pulse is 115/min, respirations are 30/min. On exam, her mucous membranes are dry. Cardiopulmonary exam is unremarkable except for tachycardia. What is the next best step in management?

   a. Urinalysis
   b. Empiric course of oral antibiotics
   c. Point-of-care blood glucose
   d. Intravenous fluids
   e. Anti-nuclear antibody
   f. No additional intervention

Test writers will use the anchoring bias to their advantage. They anticipate that everyone is vulnerable to some biases. Questions are often written intentionally to weakly suggest an incorrect diagnosis. Those who are prone to "bad" anchoring are the most vulnerable.

In prior chapters, we used the strategy of "useful, not useful, or trap." but in this case, we can focus on traps related to anchoring.

Before we read the vignette, let's review the question.

This reads:

What is the next best step in management?

Because the question does not ask for a diagnosis, we should glance at the last few sentences to see whether the diagnosis is given to us. Our inclination is to process clues and arrive at a diagnosis, but if a diagnosis is given to us, then we might be able to exert less energy while reading the vignette. This strategy is part of the 5-Step Approach detailed in Chapter 2.

In this case, a diagnosis is not stated. This means that we will have to arrive at a diagnosis and then determine the next best step in management in order to answer this question.

Now, let's read this vignette sentence by sentence. Remember, we want to focus on traps that would lead us to anchor, and clues that will lead us to the right answer. Our goal is to avoid any biases as we read the vignette.

A 17-year-old girl is brought to clinic by her mother for increased thirst and lethargy.

If we avoid "bad" anchoring, then we should consider a broad differential for increased thirst and lethargy.

What are some conditions that might cause both increased thirst and lethargy?

Diabetes mellitus or insipidus, Sjögren's syndrome, or certain medications, like anticholinergic agents, are a few possibilities.

Diabetes is a very commonly tested concept on USMLE board exams and is a likely answer choice based on probability alone. But we want to avoid anchoring on a diagnosis too early on; this would be the "bad" kind of anchoring. We can still use this as reassurance if we ultimately determine that diabetes is the most likely diagnosis, but only after we have enough information to make such a conclusion.

Over the last two days, she has become increasingly thirsty and has been urinating more frequently.

The test writer is highlighting her increased thirst again and now notes increased urination. It makes sense that someone who is drinking more fluids would urinate more than usual. It also makes sense that someone who is urinating more than usual might need to drink more to replete urinary losses. We don't know what came first.

If the test writer focuses heavily only on select information, it is easy for us to anchor on that information and neglect the entire picture. This is a test-writer strategy.

How has our differential changed with new information?

If we focus on this patient's demographics as a young female, combined with increased urination and lethargy, we might consider lupus nephritis. Other possibilities might include a urinary tract infection or, less likely, a sexually transmitted infection. But, while we could argue that increased urination might lead to increased thirst to compensate, this is usually only seen in large volume urinary losses. We would not necessarily expect such large losses with lupus or a urinary or sexually transmitted infection.

If we consider both the polydipsia and polyuria together, then the most reasonable diagnoses at this point include diabetes mellitus and diabetes insipidus. These are the only diagnoses listed as answer choices that could explain all her symptoms and should be at the top of our differential.

The mother is concerned that she has a urinary tract infection.

This sentence is designed as a trap for the anchorer. The test writer wants us to focus on her urinary symptoms. When a diagnosis is strongly alluded to like this, it is far more likely a trap than a clue. By thinking like a test writer, we should conclude from this sentence that this patient almost certainly does not have a urinary tract infection. Even so, the presence of polyuria makes the answer choice of urinalysis very tempting. Especially for the test taker that has narrowed their focus to her urinary complaints.

Her past medical history is notable for hypothyroidism and fibromyalgia.

Is there anything relevant about this medical history?

Hypothyroidism, especially in a younger female, is often a result of an autoimmune process. Autoimmune hypothyroidism often occurs with a cluster of other autoimmune diseases such as type 1 diabetes mellitus and Celiac's disease. The presence of this condition, combined with her age, might increase your concern for type 1 diabetes mellitus.

Temperature is 37 °C, blood pressure is 95/70 mmHg, pulse is 115/min, respirations are 30/min.

Vitals usually help to confirm or contradict whatever diagnosis you have anchored on.

Take a moment to think through why each of these vital signs are normal or abnormal.

Does your assessment of the vitals support your working conclusion(s)?

Generally, a fever or lack thereof will be very important in narrowing your differential. There are only a few reasons that patients will have a fever. Most commonly, these include infection or autoimmune disease, and less commonly serotonin syndrome or heat stroke.

At times, we might feel tempted to ignore information that does not fit with our conclusion, but a fever should never be ignored.

In this case, no fever is present. While the absence of fever does not exclude an infection or autoimmune disease, a normal temperature might lower this possibility on your differential.

Similarly, the absence of a fever does not exclude a urinary tract infection.

Hypotension most often suggests dehydration or shock, or can be a result of a medication side effect. Types of shock include obstructive, cardiogenic, distributive, and hypovolemic shock, as discussed in an earlier chapter.

Cardiogenic shock refers to any cardiac process that impairs the heart from pumping blood adequately through the circulation.

Obstructive shock refers to any process that physically obstructs the cardiopulmonary system from circulating blood through the circulation. This can be caused by a pulmonary embolism, pneumothorax, or cardiac tamponade.

Distributive shock refers to any process that causes vasodilation and inadequate distribution of blood throughout the body. Causes of distributive shock include sepsis, anaphylaxis, and some neurologic processes.

Hypovolemic shock refers to inadequate blood volume, rather than distribution of blood throughout the body. Causes might include severe dehydration or hemorrhage.

What systolic blood pressure is considered hypotensive?

A systolic pressure of less than 90 mmHg is considered hypotensive in adults.

But what about pediatric patients?

A good rule of thumb in pediatric patients is that the lower limit for systolic blood pressure should equal 70 + (2 x age).

Is this patient hypovolemic?

Based on our rule of thumb, the lower limit for her systolic blood pressure would equal 104 mmHg, but her systolic pressure is 95 mmHg. This pressure would classify as hypotensive, and we should be able to explain the cause with our diagnosis.

Why might this patient be hypotensive?

We know that this patient is complaining of polydipsia and polyuria. While this patient is drinking more than usual, this may still be insufficient to compensate for her excessive urination, resulting in hypovolemia.

We can consider an alternative explanation for her polyuria and polydipsia; that she has psychogenic polydipsia resulting in excessive fluid intake with consequential increased urination. But this would not explain her hypotension. Paying attention to this vital sign allows us to rule out this possibility.

Why is this patient tachycardic?

There are many possible explanations for a why a patient might be tachycardic. On board exams, the most common causes are usually cardiac, infection, dehydration, anemia, hyperthyroidism, or ingestion.

Another rule of thumb to determine whether a patient's tachycardia can be attributed solely to their fever is to add 10 bpm to their heart rate for every 1 °C above normal.

In this case, we know the patient is having excessive urinary losses, which could explain her tachycardia. None of the other common causes of tachycardia that we mentioned can explain all, or most, of her symptoms.

How do we interpret her respiratory rate?

When we are considering respiratory rate, a depressed respiratory rate on board exams only has a few common causes. These include substance ingestion, particularly opioids, respiratory fatigue from severe respiratory distress, acid-base compensation, or respiratory drive suppression by oxygen supplementation in patients with chronic carbon dioxide retention.

Tachypnea is more commonly tested on exams and is most often caused by decreased oxygen availability or acid-base disturbances.

In this case, we see that the patient is tachypneic.

What are some possible reasons why?

We have no reason to believe that she has any primary cardiopulmonary pathology. Some signs and symptoms might include shortness of breath, decreased exercise tolerance, palpitations, dizziness, syncope, or chest pain.

Can we attribute her tachypnea to an acid-base disturbance?

Earlier, we established diabetes mellitus and insipidus as two of the most likely explanations for her polyuria and polydipsia.

Can diabetes explain this patient's tachypnea?

We know from earlier chapters that diabetes mellitus can result in ketoacidosis when poorly controlled.

Can acidosis result in tachypnea?

Earlier in the text, I mentioned a trick for figuring out whether hyper- or hypoventilation will result in an increase or decrease in pH. The hyper- prefix refers to high or more, while the hypo- prefix refers to low or less. Hyperventilation will lead to a higher pH, while hypoventilation will lead to a lower pH.

If this patient was acidotic, then respiratory compensation to increase the pH would involve hyperventilation and tachypnea.

How would you summarize this patient's vitals as they relate to her clinical picture?

This patient is afebrile, mildly hypotensive, tachycardic, and tachypneic in the setting of lethargy, polydipsia, and polyuria.

We have established that her hypotension and tachycardia are most likely from excessive urinary losses, which she is attempting to compensate for with increased fluid intake. In the absence of any specific signs of cardiopulmonary pathology, her tachypnea is most likely related to an underlying acidosis. All of which can be explained by diabetes mellitus.

Let's keep reading the vignette before finalizing our conclusion(s).

On exam, her mucous membranes are dry. Cardiopulmonary exam is unremarkable except for tachycardia.

The test writer did not provide much information on physical exam, and we can gain valuable information by considering why certain findings were not included.

Recall that the test writer will always provide you with enough information to answer the question.

For example, if we expect some suprapubic tenderness in the setting of a urinary tract infection, the absence of this information in the vignette still does not exclude the possibility.

But if we were worried about a urinary tract infection or an abdominopelvic process, we would expect the test writer to at least mention an abdominal exam was performed. While this is not an absolute rule, the absence of an abdominopelvic exam in general should decrease your suspicion for an abdominopelvic process.

In this case, the test writer did not mention an abdominal exam. This should lower our suspicion for a urinary tract infection.

This vignette was designed to weakly suggest a renal or urinary tract pathology. Those prone to anchoring might focus on renal or urinary tract causes of her symptoms.

As discussed earlier, diabetes mellitus is the only condition that would explain her polydipsia, polyuria, lethargy, dehydration, and tachypnea. This should be the diagnosis we "good" anchor on at this point.

Now that we have a diagnosis, let's review the answer choices.

As a reminder, the answer choices read:

a. *Urinalysis*
b. *Empiric course of oral antibiotics*
c. *Point-of-care blood glucose*
d. *Intravenous fluids*
e. *Anti-nuclear antibody*
f. *No additional intervention*

Though we should no longer be suspicious for urinary tract or renal pathology at this point, a urinalysis may still be a tempting answer choice. A urinalysis could reveal whether glucose and/or ketones are present, which would help to confirm our diagnosis of DKA.

There are two reasons to not pick urinalysis as the correct answer.

First, what pathology and/or diagnosis is alluded to with a urinalysis?

This answer choice targets those who are suspicious of a renal and/or urinary tract pathology. But, because a urinalysis can still provide us with information about a patient's hydration status and hyperglycemia, this might be a tempting answer choice.

Second, what is the best first step in diagnosing DKA?

A point-of-care blood glucose is the first step in making this diagnosis. If the blood glucose is 150, then DKA is less likely. But if the glucose level is 300 or 400, then we might feel more confident in our diagnosis and initiate treatment sooner.

Keep in mind, the presence of high blood glucose alone cannot diagnose DKA. Many diabetic patients have high glucose levels but are not in a state of ketoacidosis.

Regardless of whether this patient is in DKA or not, the initial treatment based on a high point-of-care glucose is very similar. Treatment is focused on stabilizing blood glucose, electrolytes, and rehydration.

If one element of treatment is rehydration, then why is the correct answer not intravenous fluids?

This answer choice is another trap for the anchorer. The test writers have put a lot of emphasis on this patient's dehydration. If we had not taken the time to consider why this patient is dehydrated, then we might feel inclined to select this answer.

There is an argument for starting intravenous fluids first. This patient is clearly dehydrated with abnormal vital signs.

How do you choose between a point-of-care glucose and intravenous fluids?

In reality, you would not really have this dilemma in the hospital. Both would happen simultaneously.

But this question is designed to test your ability to identify the diagnosis and the best treatment course.

If we were to administer fluids without treating the underlying problem, how much would our patient improve?

Without addressing the underlying problem, this patient would continue to have excessive urinary losses. This is like putting a band aid on a hemorrhaging wound.

Keep in mind that there is nothing to prevent this patient from drinking by mouth. Despite polydipsia, she is unable to maintain euvolemia. IV fluids alone would not be much more effective.

What is the best choice to manage her dehydration?

We know that her polyuria is from osmotic diuresis, and she will continue to lose fluids excessively until her diabetes is addressed. By treating her diabetes, she should no longer continue to have excessive losses.

One trick I often teach students is that the correct answer is almost always normal saline, though not in this case. While not applicable here, any answer choice that mentions normal saline should be strongly considered. This will more commonly be true in questions that ask about what the best fluid choice is to administer.

In reviewing the other answer choices, we can exclude anti-nuclear antibody based on our low suspicion of autoimmune process, as well as empiric course of oral antibiotics given the absence of fever.

Finally, let's consider the possibility of "no additional intervention."

This answer choice commonly results in second guessing and self-doubt. It is strategic for test writers to include. Often, it is the correct answer. But just as often, it isn't.

If a patient has abnormal vital signs, you should almost certainly recommend some type of intervention.

Recall that we do not need to be able to exclude answer choices to feel confident in our answer choice and move on to the next question.

What is the correct answer?

Point-of-care blood glucose

In the real world, a point-of-care blood glucose and fluids would be ordered simultaneously along with a basic metabolic panel. Within 30 minutes, we would have made a diagnosis and initiated treatment. But remember, questions are designed to test specific knowledge. In this case, the test writer wants to test your understanding of diabetes management and pathophysiology and can do this with what might feel like an artificial scenario.

Despite various traps laid out by the test writer, we were able to arrive at a diagnosis that could explain all of the major clinical features in the vignette and an answer choice that seemed most reasonable given our knowledge and reasoning skills.

Question 2

A 12-year-old Asian male presents to clinic with joint pain and rash. His mother noticed a rash over his legs and trunk for the past few days. The patient has also been complaining of joint pain. His initial knee and ankle pain have resolved, but this morning he woke up with wrist and elbow pain. The patient has been healthy except for a recent upper respiratory illness several weeks ago that has since resolved. He denies any ocular symptoms, emesis, diarrhea, or urinary symptoms. In clinic, his temperature is found to be 38.5 °C, pulse is 77/min, and respirations are 16/min. Physical exam is notable for stiff and tender wrist joints bilaterally. There is a pink, well demarcated, nonpruritic rash over the trunk and lower extremities. EKG demonstrates a slightly prolonged PR interval. Which of the following is the most likely diagnosis?

a. Systemic juvenile idiopathic arthritis
b. Lyme disease
c. Acute rheumatic fever
d. Kawasaki disease
e. Reactive arthritis
f. Henoch-Schönlein purpura

Let's first address ethnicity as it relates to board exams.

Board exam questions will often associate certain diseases with a particular ethnicity. Examiners tend to include ethnicity as part of the vignette in two scenarios; either to lead you to the correct answer or anchor you to the wrong one.

We should never prematurely anchor on a diagnosis or ignore a potential diagnosis because of these associations.

Can you think of some common associations made by examiners?

African American: Systemic lupus erythematous, sarcoidosis, sickle cell disease

Asian American: Kawasaki disease, Takayasu's arteritis

Latin American Immigrant: Rheumatic fever, Chagas disease

Asian or Latin American Immigrant: Tuberculosis

African Immigrant: Malaria, sickle cell disease

Mediterranean descent: Thalassemia, glucose-6-phosphate dehydrogenase deficiency

Ashkenazi Jew: Tay-Sachs disease, cystic fibrosis

It is important to highlight that these associations have been criticized as problematic in real world settings. While associating diseases with certain ethnicities can be useful in some cases, the bias that these associations create can lead to missed diagnoses and inequities in medical care.

There are numerous examples of improper medical care due to these associations. One historic example is the baseless belief that Black or African American patients feel less pain and thus require less analgesia.

Another example that I encountered in medical school was a pediatric patient who underwent extensive work up for recurrent pneumonias, though the diagnosis remained elusive for many years. No one thought to test him for cystic fibrosis until he was almost 3 or 4 years old.

Did the fact that this patient was African American delay the diagnosis, despite having had an otherwise classic presentation?

In school, we are taught to associate Cystic Fibrosis with Caucasian ethnicity and Ashkenazi Jewish background. But as this example highlights, if our training over-emphasizes the importance of race and/or ethnicity, then we are more likely to miss a diagnosis. This is a perfect example of the "bad" kind of anchoring.

Always remember to use demographic information cautiously. Ethnicity and/or race will probably be more useful on board exams than in real life.

If you are someone that picks up on patterns, then you will likely benefit from noting the patterns board examiners use in association with race. But patterns are not absolute, and you should never solely rely on them.

In fact, if you are prone to premature anchoring, you may benefit from ignoring race altogether on exams. Knowledge of race and/or ethnicity will never be necessary to answer a question, only helpful.

Let's return to the practice question.

From the perspective of test-taking strategy, we can assign importance to the fact that the test writer included Asian ethnicity in the vignette.

We need to decide whether the mention of ethnicity is designed to anchor you to the wrong diagnosis or to direct you to the right one.

What did we learn from the first sentence?

We learn that this is an Asian patient with joint pain and rash.

What types of medical conditions will cause joint pain and rash?

Joint pain and rash should make us think of infection or autoimmune disease.

Are there any infectious and/or autoimmune diseases that are commonly associated with Asian race on board exams?

Kawasaki disease should come to mind (Figure 5-1).

From this point, we can read the rest of the vignette with the perspective that the test writer might want us to think about Kawasaki disease based on the mention of Asian ethnicity. But we do not know yet whether this will be the correct or the incorrect answer.

Let's read the rest of the vignette from the perspective that the diagnosis is indeed Kawasaki disease. This should help to illustrate how anchoring can shift perspective.

His mother noticed a rash over his legs and trunk for the past few days. The patient has also been complaining of joint pain. His initial knee and ankle pain have resolved, but this morning he woke up with wrist and elbow pain.

We already know this patient had a rash and joint pain. This information provides further details but does not provide much new information. Nothing so far seems to contradict our diagnosis of Kawasaki disease.

The patient has been healthy except for a recent upper respiratory illness several weeks ago that has since resolved.

What is the significance of a recent upper respiratory illness?

Perhaps this recent illness precipitated Kawasaki disease.

He denies any ocular symptoms, emesis, diarrhea, or urinary symptoms.

Does this new information contradict our diagnosis of Kawasaki disease?

While the presence of ocular symptoms like conjunctivitis might support a diagnosis of Kawasaki disease, the absence is not necessarily contradictory.

In clinic, his temperature is found to be 38.5 °C (101.3 °F), pulse is 77/min, and respirations are 16/min.

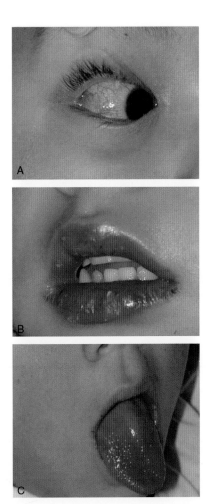

FIGURE 5-1 Physical Exam Findings in Kawasaki Disease. Key physical exam findings in Kawasaki disease include (**A**) conjunctivitis, (**B**) mucositis, and (**C**) "strawberry tongue." Other findings include a rash and hand/foot swelling. (Reproduced with permission from Shah SS, Kemper AR, Ratner AJ. *Pediatric Infectious Diseases: Essentials for Practice*, 2nd ed. McGraw Hill, 2019.)

What information is provided by these vital signs?

The patient is febrile, but his vital signs are otherwise normal. A fever can be seen in both an infectious or an autoimmune process.

Physical exam is notable for stiff and tender wrist joints bilaterally. There is a pink, well demarcated, nonpruritic rash over the trunk and lower extremities.

Could we expect these findings in Kawasaki disease?

Joint pain and rash are both features of Kawasaki disease.

EKG demonstrates a slightly prolonged PR interval.

Is there cardiac involvement in Kawasaki disease?

There is!

Notice how we are conforming new information to fit with our diagnosis, rather than allowing the new information to direct us.

At what points in the vignette should we have paused to consider other diagnoses?

The patient has been healthy except for a recent upper respiratory illness several weeks ago that has since resolved.

While Kawasaki disease might be precipitated by upper respiratory symptoms, we should have paused to consider other possibilities. Examples might include acute rheumatic fever or Guillain-Barre syndrome.

There is a pink, well demarcated, nonpruritic rash over the trunk and lower extremities.

This is a fairly specific description for a rash. The most generic description for a pediatric rash is typically a maculopapular rash over the trunk and extremities.

Can you think of some other rash descriptions or "buzz words" that are specific to disease processes?

Sandpaper-like rash is used to describe acute rheumatic fever (Figure 5-2A). Well-demarcated, pink rash can refer to erysipelas (Figure 5-2B). Rash involving the hands and soles refers to Hand, foot, and mouth disease (Figure 5-3), rickettsia infection, or syphilis. Vesicles suggest any type of herpesvirus (Figure 5-4). Yellow crusting on the face describes impetigo (Figure 5-2C). Umbilicated papules suggest molluscum contagiosum (Figure 5-5).

Unfortunately, we cannot remember the disease processes for every rash. But we can at least recognize that a specific disease process is being referenced in this description.

We should consider whether the typical rash in Kawasaki disease would or could be described by this type of rash.

What is the typical rash seen in Henoch-Schönlein purpura (HSP)?

This rash is typically a palpable purpuric rash over the buttocks and lower extremities (Figure 5-6). The description of a well demarcated rash over the lower extremities could theoretically describe the typical rash seen in HSP. Combined with the age and gender of this patient, HSP is also a tempting diagnosis to anchor on.

But, while similar, the description of this rash does not quite fit with the typical rash we see in HSP. Just as we are trying to do with Kawasaki, we should avoid prematurely anchoring on or conforming new information to the diagnosis of HSP.

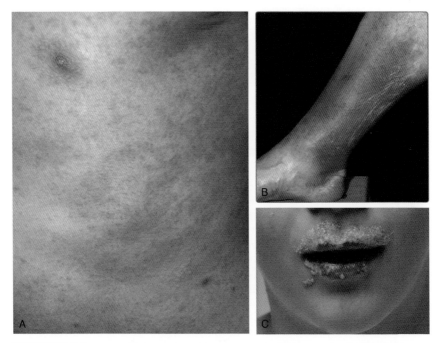

FIGURE 5-2 Rashes Seen in Group A *Streptococcus* Infection. (A) Acute Rheumatic Fever. "Sandpaper" rash is the hallmark rash seen in acute rheumatic fever. The rash has been described to feel like "sandpaper", thus the name. (B) Erysipelas. Erysipelas is a skin infection like cellulitis, except that it affects the more superficial layers of the skin. This rash is typically described to have "well demarcated borders." Most often, these infections are caused by Group A streptococcal bacteria. (C) Impetigo. Impetigo is a common skin infection that is characterized by its "honey crust" lesions. The rash is usually erythematous with a yellow-brown crust overlying the area. The face and mouth are common locations for this infection. (A: Used with permission from Richard P. Usatine, MD. From Usatine RP, et al. *The Color Atlas & Synopsis of Family Medicine*, 3rd ed. McGraw Hill, 2019. B: Reproduced with permission from Kang S, et al. *Fitzpatrick's Dermatology*, 9th ed. McGraw Hill, 2019. C: Reproduced with permission from Tenenbein M, et al. *Strange and Schafermeyer's Pediatric Emergency Medicine*, 5th ed. McGraw Hill, 2019.)

EKG demonstrates a slightly prolonged PR interval (Figure 5-7).

Does this EKG finding support the diagnosis of Kawasaki disease?

It's true that there is cardiac involvement in Kawasaki disease.

But what is the cardiac involvement seen in Kawasaki disease?

Kawasaki disease can lead to coronary artery aneurysmal dilation. This is why these patients take aspirin, despite the increased risk of Reye's syndrome in the pediatric population. Remember that aspirin is otherwise avoided in this population because of this risk.

While we may not know whether a prolonged PR interval is also a feature of Kawasaki disease, we should be cautious about using this finding as support

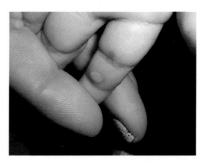

FIGURE 5-3 Hand, Foot, and Mouth Disease. Hand, foot, and mouth disease is a viral illness causing typical symptoms such as fever and sore throat. The hallmark feature of this illness is the rash involving the mouth, hands, and feet, particularly the palms and soles. The rash can include erythematous macules and/or vesicles. (Used with permission from Richard P. Usatine, MD. From Usatine RP, Smith MA, Mayeaux EJ Jr, Chumley HS. *The Color Atlas & Synopsis of Family Medicine*, 3rd ed. McGraw Hill, 2019.)

of Kawasaki disease simply because it suggests cardiac involvement. Not all cardiac involvement is created equal.

These findings—the rash, the cardiac disease—are similar, but not a perfect fit, to the features we know are present in Kawasaki disease.

When the test writer is careful to avoid including any major red flags, such as is the case here, we become even more vulnerable to anchoring. But, if we are careful, we should notice that there are enough features in the vignette that don't perfectly fit with Kawasaki disease.

When we are careful to avoid anchoring, we are also more likely to pick up on what supporting evidence *isn't* included in the vignette.

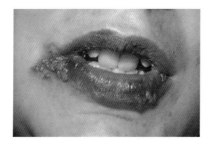

FIGURE 5-4 Herpes Labialis. Herpes labialis is a herpetic infection of the lips. The hallmark of herpes labialis is the presence of vesicles involving the "vermillion border." Vesicles may be described as a dew drop on a rose petal because the vesicle typically overlies an erythematous base. (Reproduced with permission from Soutor C, Hordinsky MK. *Clinical Dermatology*. McGraw Hill, 2013.)

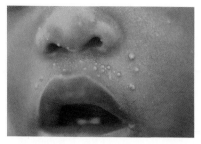

FIGURE 5-5 Molluscum Contagiosum. Molluscum contagiosum is a benign, mild skin infection. The rash typically presents as round, flesh-colored papules with an umbilicated center. They may present anywhere on the body and are sometimes associated with itching. (Reproduced with permission from Soutor C, Hordinsky MK. *Clinical Dermatology.* McGraw Hill, 2013.)

What is the typical presentation you might expect for Kawasaki disease?

You might expect a fever and joint pain, maculopapular rash on the trunk, erythematous hands and feet, mucositis, and/or conjunctivitis.

In the case of this vignette, we have the fever, joint pain, and rash only. And these features are common in a number of disease processes, not just Kawasaki disease.

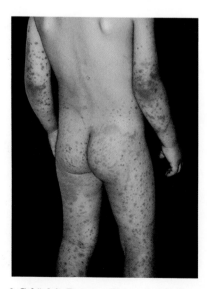

FIGURE 5-6 Henoch-Schönlein Purpura. The typical rash seen in patients with Henoch-Schönlein purpura is described as a "palpable" purpura. The most classic distribution involves the buttocks and lower extremities. (Photo contributor: Kevin J. Knoop, MD, MS from Knoop KJ, Stack LB, Storrow AB, Thurman RJ. *The Atlas of Emergency Medicine,* 5th ed. McGraw Hill, 2021.)

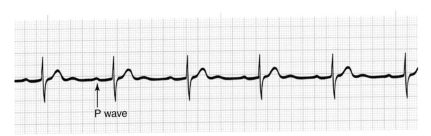

FIGURE 5-7 Prolonged PR Interval on EKG. It is defined by a PR interval greater than 200 milliseconds, equivalent to the size of one big box on a rhythm strip. This represents excessive conduction delay at the AV node. (Reproduced with permission from DeTurk WE, Cahalin LP. *Cardiovascular and Pulmonary Physical Therapy: An Evidence-Based Approach*, 3rd ed. McGraw Hill, 2018.)

Let's read the vignette again, now using a more methodical approach and avoiding anchoring.

There are many different approaches we could use for this question. Given that we know this patient has vague symptoms that might suggest a number of diagnoses, we will likely benefit from reviewing the answer choices as a way to guide our focus.

As a reminder, the answer choices are:

  a. *Systemic juvenile idiopathic arthritis*
  b. *Lyme disease*
  c. *Acute rheumatic fever*
  d. *Kawasaki disease*
  e. *Reactive arthritis*
  f. *Henoch-Schönlein purpura*

We can keep these diagnoses in mind as we read through the vignette again.

A 12-year-old Asian boy presents to clinic with joint pain and rash.

Joint pain and rash seem concerning for an autoimmune process or infection of some kind. Asian ethnicity might increase suspicion for Kawasaki disease.

His mother noticed a rash over his legs and trunk for the past few days.

The mention of the past few days suggests that this is an acute process. An autoimmune condition is more likely to have slower progression, which might decrease the likelihood of systemic juvenile idiopathic arthritis.

Notice that we are adjusting the likelihood of one diagnosis over another, without anchoring prematurely on a single diagnosis.

The patient has also been complaining of joint pain. His initial knee and ankle pain have resolved, but this morning he woke up with wrist and elbow pain.

Rather than generalizing this information as "joint pain," let's synthesize this information to determine whether there is anything more specific and helpful within these sentences.

By noting that the patient first had knee and ankle pain, which resolved, and now has new wrist and elbow pain, the test writer is describing a migratory polyarthritis.

With what conditions do we see migratory polyarthritis?

Migratory polyarthritis is a feature of Lyme disease, acute rheumatic fever, and Henoch–Schönlein purpura.

The patient has been healthy except for a recent upper respiratory illness several weeks ago that has since resolved.

If we assume that this upper respiratory illness precipitated this patient's current illness, then a diagnosis of Lyme disease or systemic juvenile idiopathic arthritis would seem less likely.

He denies any ocular symptoms, emesis, diarrhea, or urinary symptoms.

Ocular symptoms are often present in Kawasaki disease, though not a requirement. Urinary symptoms might be present in Henoch–Schönlein purpura from IgA nephritis, but not necessary either.

In clinic, his temperature is found to be 38.5 °C (101.3 °F), pulse is 77/min, and respirations are 16/min.

This is a relatively high fever that might be seen in diseases such as Kawasaki disease or acute rheumatic fever.

At this point, the key features that we have highlighted include the presence of a migratory polyarthritis and a high fever. These are features that we missed earlier when we had prematurely anchored on Kawasaki disease.

Physical exam is notable for stiff and tender wrist joints bilaterally. There is a pink, well demarcated, nonpruritic rash over the trunk and lower extremities.

You may notice that the mention of a well demarcated rash over the lower extremities is designed to lure you into choosing HSP, despite not perfectly fitting with what you may know about that rash.

The rash description is actually most consistent with acute rheumatic fever. However, you do not need to know this to answer the question.

EKG demonstrates a slightly prolonged PR interval.

What disease is described by a prolonged PR interval?

A prolonged PR interval is first degree heart block.

If we anchored on this finding in isolation, we might be tempted to choose Lyme disease. However, there were many features in the vignette that suggest Lyme disease is not the correct answer. We should remind ourselves of this even when a single finding comes up that might strongly suggest a diagnosis.

We can protect ourselves by considering the entire presentation and remaining weary of test-writer traps.

At this point, acute rheumatic fever is our leading diagnosis because of the fever, precipitating illness, and migratory polyarthritis.

What is a typical presentation of acute rheumatic fever?

Some of us may recall the JONES criteria. (Figure 5-8). This is the major criteria for diagnosing acute rheumatic fever.

What does JONES stand for?

J for joints (migratory polyarthritis), O for heart (myocarditis), N for nodules, E for erythema marginatum, and S for Sydenham chorea.

What are the minor criteria for diagnosing acute rheumatic fever?

The minor criteria are less memorable, but include PR prolongation, arthralgias, CRP/ESR elevation, and fever.

Major Criteria	Minor Criteria
J: Joints (signs of arthritis typically involving knees, ankles, elbows, wrists)	Fever
O: Carditis (involvement can include endocardium, myocardium, epicardium, pericardium)	Arthralgias (if not using arthritis as a major criteria)
N: Subcutaneous Nodules (painless firm nodules over bones)	Prolonged PR interval
E: Erythema Marginatum (well demarcated nonpuritic rash over trunk and extending to extremities)	Acute phase reactants: elevated WBC, CRP, ESR
S: Sydenham Chorea (abrupt purposeless movements, when present is diagnostic)	Previous diagnosis of rheumatic fever

FIGURE 5-8 Major and Minor Criteria for Acute Rheumatic Fever. The presence of two major criteria or one major and two minor criteria in the setting of prior streptococcal infection is required for a diagnosis of acute rheumatic fever. (Reproduced with permission from Shah SS, Ludwig S. *Symptom-Based Diagnosis in Pediatrics.* McGraw Hill, 2014.)

What features that are typical for acute rheumatic fever are present in this vignette?

We see migratory polyarthritis, a mysterious rash that could describe erythema marginatum, a fever, and PR prolongation. We also have a history of prior upper respiratory illness that might represent an untreated Strep B infection.

What is the correct answer?

Acute rheumatic fever

We methodically went through the vignette the second time and used new information to adjust the likelihood of a given diagnosis. As we narrowed our differential diagnoses, we considered what features we should expect a test writer to include if they expected us to confidently select one answer choice over the others. This approach allowed us to arrive at an answer that we may have otherwise not even considered. Without going through this process methodically, we easily could have anchored on one of the incorrect answer choices.

Question 3

A 10-year-old girl presents to clinic for headache following a bicycle accident that occurred a few hours earlier. She was bicycling alongside her mother when she lost her balance as she made a turn. The patient fell and struck her head and knee on the ground. She did not lose consciousness. She subsequently developed mild nausea without emesis and head pain localized to the area of impact. Vitals and neurologic exam were normal. The patient appeared uncomfortable during the abdominal exam and scopolamine was prescribed for nausea. The patient presents to the emergency room the following day for agitation. Her parents report that she started acting strangely a few hours earlier and has seemed increasingly agitated. Medical history is only significant for allergies, which are well managed with diphenhydramine. Temperature is 37.9 °C, blood pressure is 125/80 mmHg, pulse is 160/min, respirations are 22/min. She is pacing during the exam and is not cooperative with answering questions. Pupils are equal and 7 mm bilaterally. Extraocular movements are intact. Facial movements are symmetric. Mucous membranes are dry. Cardiac exam is notable for tachycardia. Abdominal exam is notable for decreased bowel sounds and a palpable mass in the lower abdomen with mild tenderness to palpation. The remainder of the exam is normal. Which of the following is the best next step in management of this patient?

a. Head CT
b. Brain MRI
c. Lumbar puncture
d. Physostigmine
e. Mannitol
f. Emergency surgery
g. Psychiatry consultation

Let's first review the first and the last two sentences of the vignette so that we can better establish the context.

This reads:

A 10-year-old girl presents to clinic for headache following a bicycle accident that occurred a few hours earlier. She was bicycling alongside her mother when she lost her balance as she made a turn.

The remainder of the exam is normal. Which of the following is the best next step in management of this patient?

How would we summarize this vignette based on this information?

A 10-year-old girl presents to clinic for headache after falling off her bicycle. What is the best next step in management of this patient?

What do you think are some reasonable next steps based on our summary?

A headache following a bicycle accident is not unusual and may represent pain from local trauma or from a concussion. Both scenarios do not require imaging, and the next best step would be supportive care.

On the otherhand, if this patient demonstrated any signs concerning for an intracranial bleed, such as focal neurological findings, altered mental status, or loss of consciousness, emergent imaging would be indicated.

If pain or abnormal physical exam findings related to her extremities or abdomen are noted, then appropriate imaging might be indicated. However, this would likely be less emergent than head imaging, unless there is concern for hemodynamic instability related to internal hemorrhage. However, given the mechanism of the injury, this is highly unlikely.

Now that we have generated a framework for this scenario, we can proceed with reviewing the answer choices.

In reviewing the answer choices, we need to remember that this question requires us to both establish the diagnosis and then determine the next best step. Because of this, it may be most helpful to work backwards from the answer choices to arrive at a diagnosis and answer this question confidently.

As we begin to identify one or a few diagnoses that we would associate with each answer choice, think of some features that you might expect in the vignette that would lead you to choose that answer.

As a reminder, the answer choices read:

a. *Head CT scan*
b. *Brain MRI*
c. *Lumbar puncture*

d. *Physostigmine*
e. *Mannitol*
f. *Emergency surgery*
g. *Psychiatry consultation*

Can you identify the "trap" answer choice(s) if you were to "bad" anchor?

When a test writer overly emphasizes a point, then you should become suspicious of the test writer's motives.

While the head injury is not necessarily overly emphasized in this case, it is certainly emphasized. Whether this is the appropriate focal point, or a trap, is to be determined.

If the head injury is indeed a trap, then anchoring too heavily on the head injury will steer us in the wrong direction. And visa versa.

We can also evaluate the answer choices and determine some of the directions that the test writer expects us to go.

Answers a, b, c, e, and f refer to a head injury (+/− lumbar puncture). Based on the rules of probability, choosing one of these options seems like a good bet.

What do the other answer choices tell us?

The test writer will not include answer choices that are obviously incorrect. There should always be a reason that an answer choice was included.

Physostigmine and psychiatric consultation (+/− lumbar puncture) are the only answers that seem unrelated to her head injury. Given this, we should consider why the test writer included these choices.

Let's evaluate the answer choices in more detail to see if we can determine why particular answer choices were included.

How might you assign diagnoses to each answer choice?

Head CT scan

A head CT is commonly used in cases of trauma or stroke. CT is a fast and effective imaging modality for the diagnosis of intracranial hemorrhage. For ischemic stroke, MRI is the best form of imaging but can take longer than a head CT in many hospitals, which is why head CT is typically first line for an acute stroke evaluation. While CT imaging is faster, this will not detect an ischemic stroke in the early stages.

Do you recall the four major categories for intracranial hemorrhage?

These include epidural (Figure 5-9), subdural (Figure 5-10), subarachnoid (Figure 5-11), and intraparenchymal (Figure 5-12) hemorrhages.

The most emergent bleed that results from head trauma is taught as the epidural hemorrhage.

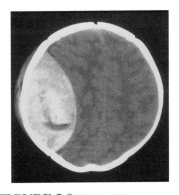

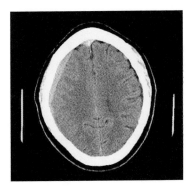

FIGURE 5-9 Epidural Hematoma.
Epidural hematoma can be identified
by its classic biconvex shape. This is
because hemorrhage in the epidural space
cannot expand beyond the suture lines.
(Reproduced with permission from Brust
JCM. *CURRENT Diagnosis & Treatment:
Neurology*, 3rd ed. McGraw Hill, 2019.)

FIGURE 5-10 Subdural Hematoma.
Subdural hematoma can be classified by
its crescent shape. A subdural hematoma
will not be confined by suture lines.
(Reproduced with permission from
Rozenfeld RA. *The PICU Handbook.*
McGraw Hill, 2018.)

How does epidural hemorrhage present?

This classically presents as a loss of consciousness followed by a lucid phase, and then deterioration of mental status up to recurrent loss of consciousness. If the patient loses consciousness again, the outcome tends to be poor.

How does subdural hemorrhage present?

Subdural hemorrhage is less often tested. Some testable scenarios include an infant with non-accidental trauma with retinal hemorrhages on exam, or an elderly patient with a fall and insidious onset of symptoms over several weeks.

How does subarachnoid hemorrhage present?

Subarachnoid hemorrhage is typically associated with an older adult with hypertension or aneurysms. These hemorrhages are associated with the "worst headache" or "thunderclap headache."

How does intraparenchymal hemorrhage present?

Intraparenchymal hemorrhage is less commonly tested and refers to any bleed in the intraparenchymal space. This represents a broad category, and can have multiple causes such as hypertension, aneurysms, tumor, or injury.

If we are considering intracranial bleed as a possibility, then we should recall the most common signs and symptoms.

Many of the symptoms related to intracranial bleeds have to do with increased intracranial pressure. Recall that the intracranial space is not expandable. Any bleed will lead to increased pressure as the intracranial contents fight for space.

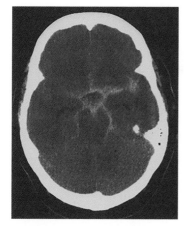

FIGURE 5-11 Subarachnoid Hemorrhage. Recall that the subarachnoid space is filled with cerebrospinal fluid. In the case of a subarachnoid hemorrhage, the spaces that typically appear black when filled with cerebrospinal fluid should appear grayer as they fill with blood. (Reproduced with permission from Malone TR, Hazle C, Grey ML. *Imaging in Rehabilitation.* McGraw Hill, 2008.)

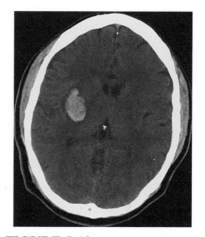

FIGURE 5-12 Intraparenchymal Hemorrhage. Intraparenchymal hemorrhage is any bleed that occurs within the brain parenchyma. Brain parenchyma includes the cerebrum and the ventricles. (Reproduced with permission from Amthor FR, Theibert AB, Standaert DG, Roberson ED. *Essentials of Modern Neuroscience.* McGraw Hill, 2020.)

Classic symptoms of increased intracranial pressure include headache or papilledema. A highly testable concept is the "blown pupil(s)" seen when the brain herniates and compresses cranial nerve III, resulting in dilated pupils that are not responsive to light.

Let's continue with the other answer choices.

Brain MRI

We know that MRI is an imaging modality that provides more detail than CT, but at the expense of time. Because of timing, MRI is typically not used in emergent scenarios.

Can you think of some common scenarios where MRI is used?

MRI is used for diagnosis of intracranial masses, such as abscesses or tumors. Other intracranial findings such as calcifications, demyelination, or tubers are also visualized on MRI.

While MRI is a great imaging modality to diagnose stroke, the timing of MRI often precludes this as first line.

In considering whether brain MRI is the correct answer, we should consider the diagnosis we are concerned about.

If we are highly suspicious of an intracranial bleed, then head CT should be our first-line tool for evaluation.

MRI would only be the correct answer in a non-emergent case requiring more detailed visualization of the brain.

Given what we know so far about the clinical scenario, this answer seems unlikely to be the correct choice.

Lumbar puncture

What is the most common diagnostic category evaluated by lumbar puncture?

Lumbar puncture is most often used to evaluate for infection (Figure 5-13).

Lumbar puncture can also be used to evaluate for other diagnoses, such as autoimmune conditions affecting the CNS, though this is less common.

If lumbar puncture was the correct answer, we would most likely see signs of infection such as fever, headache, neck stiffness, and possibly altered mental status. We may even see petechiae in the case of a *N. meningitidis* infection.

Physostigmine

Diagnosis	Appearance	Opening Pressure (mm H_2O)	WBC (per mcL); Differential	RBC (per mcL)	CSF Glucose (mg/dL)	CSF Protein (mg/dL)	CSF Culture
Normal	Clear, colorless	70-200	≤5 mononuclear cells; 0 polymorphonuclear neutrophils	0	45-85 (or 2/3 serum)	15-45	Negative
Bacterial meningitis	Cloudy	↑↑↑↑	200–20,000; mostly polymorphonuclear neutrophils (>80%)	0	<45 (or CSF:serum glucose ratio ≤0.4)	>50	Positive
Viral (aseptic) meningitis	Normal	Normal or ↑	100-1000; mostly mononuclear cells	0	45-85	Normal or ↑	Negative
Mycobacterial (tuberculous) meningitis	Normal or cloudy	↑↑↑	100-1000; mostly mononuclear cells	0	<45	>50	±
Fungal meningitis	Normal or cloudy	Normal or ↑	100-1000; mostly mononuclear cells		<45	>50	±

FIGURE 5-13 CSF Analysis for Central Nervous System Infections. Differences in cell count can help to determine whether a bacterial, viral, mycobacterial, or fungal meningitis is present. (Reproduced with permission from Sutton SS. *McGraw Hill's NAPLEX®Review Guide,* 4th ed. McGraw Hill, 2021.)

What is the mechanism of physostigmine?

Physostigmine is a cholinesterase inhibitor that is primarily used in the case of anticholinergic poisoning or toxicity.

When I was memorizing drugs for pharmacology, I made up a general rule that drugs ending in "mine" were antagonists or inhibitors. This is because *mean* people will *antagonize* you (Figure 5-14).

This works for some of the basic alpha antagonists like phentolamine and phenoxybenzamine, as well as the cholinesterase/acetylcholinesterase antagonists like rivastigmine and physostigmine.

Though all are "antagonists," there is an important distinction to be made. While drugs like phentolamine antagonize or inhibit alpha receptors, thereby decreasing sympathetic activity, drugs like physostigmine antagonize or inhibit

Drug	Action	Clinical Applications
Direct-Acting Agonists		
Bethanechol (muscarinic)	Activates bowel and bladder smooth muscle	Postoperative and neurogenic ileus and urinary retention
Nicotine (nicotinic)	Replaces rapid-onset actions (cigarette) with slower action	Smoking deterrence (patch, chewing gum)
Indirect-Acting Agonists		
Neostigmine (carbamate) Pyridostigmine (carbamate) Edrophonium (alcohol)	Amplifies effects of endogenous ACh	Treatment of myasthenia gravis Reversal of neuromuscular blockade by nondepolarizing drugs
Physostigmine (carbamate) Echothiophate (organophosphate)	Amplifies effects of endogenous ACh	Glaucoma
Donepezil (atypical) Galantaine (atypical) Rivastigmine (carbamate)	Amplifies effects of endogenous ACh in the CNS	Alzheimer's disease

FIGURE 5-14 Cholinergic Medications. (Reproduced with permission from Jobst EE, Panus PC, Kruidering-Hall M. *Pharmacology for the Physical Therapist*, 2nd ed. McGraw Hill, 2020.)

the enzyme that breaks down acetylcholine, thereby increasing acetylcholine availability and enhancing cholinergic activity.

Can you think of some of the clinical uses of physostigmine?

Physostigmine is a cholinesterase inhibitor that is primarily used in the case of anticholinergic poisoning or toxicity.

Can you think of some of the clinical uses of rivastigmine?

Acetylcholinesterase inhibitors like donepazil, rivastigmine, and galantamine are used for conditions that affect memory, such as Alzheimer's dementia.

Unlike physostigmine, the acetylcholinesterase inhibitors used for conditions affecting memory are uncommonly tested after the USMLE Step 1 exam. If you feel inclined to memorize them, there is a mnemonic you can use;

A *galant* gentleman rescued a *damsel* in distress by the *river*.

Galant sounds like *galantamine, damsel* sounds like *donepazil*, and *river* sounds like *rivastigmine.*

If physostigmine is indeed the correct answer, then we should expect to see signs of anticholinergic toxicity such as an exaggerated sympathetic nervous system response. There should also be clues suggesting ingestion of an anticholinergic agent or agents.

What clinical presentation might suggest an exaggerated sympathetic nervous system response?

When in doubt, consider the differences between "fight or flight," the sympathetic response, and "rest and digest," the parasympathetic response (Figure 5-15).

For the "fight or flight" response, consider running from a bear.

Your anxiety levels would likely increase, maintaining hypervigilance during the chase. You need to visualize your surroundings, and pupillary dilation will allow you to do so at the sacrifice of visual acuity. And it would be a disaster if, while running from a bear, you suddenly needed to use the bathroom, so urinary retention is quite useful in this instance. And you will want to preserve energy for running from the bear, so digesting your last meal can wait.

This describes the sympathetic response.

The opposite is true for the "rest and digest" response.

Consider sitting on a sofa by the fire reading a good book. You will need better visual acuity to read, and so your pupils might constrict. Your surroundings are less important in this instance. As you read your book by the fire, your anxiety levels decrease. Since you are relaxed, your body has plenty of energy to digest your food and you have ample opportunities to use the bathroom.

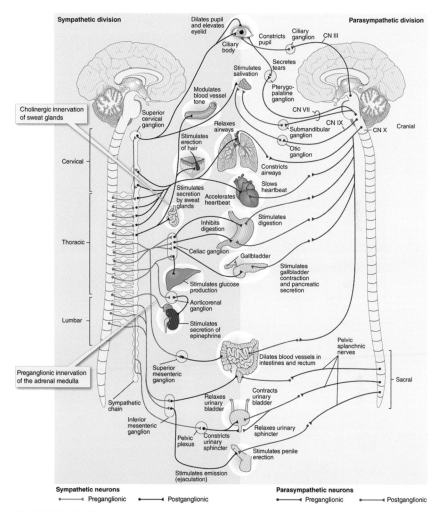

Sympathetic division

Dilates pupil and elevates eyelid

Ciliary body

Constricts pupil

Ciliary ganglion   CN III

Parasympathetic division

Stimulates salivation

Secretes tears

Pterygo-palatine ganglion

Cholinergic innervation of sweat glands

Modulates blood vessel tone

CN VII

CN IX

Submandibular ganglion

CN X

Cranial

Superior cervical ganglion

Relaxes airways

Stimulates erection of hair

Otic ganglion

Cervical

Constricts airways

Stimulates secretion by sweat glands

Accelerates heartbeat

Slows heartbeat

Inhibits digestion

Stimulates digestion

Thoracic

Celiac ganglion

Gallbladder

Stimulates gallbladder contraction and pancreatic secretion

Stimulates glucose production

Aorticorenal ganglion

Lumbar

Stimulates secretion of epinephrine

Pelvic splanchnic nerves

Dilates blood vessels in intestines and rectum

Sacral

Superior mesenteric ganglion

Preganglionic innervation of the adrenal medulla

Contracts urinary bladder

Sympathetic chain

Relaxes urinary bladder

Inferior mesenteric ganglion

Relaxes urinary sphincter

Pelvic plexus

Constricts urinary sphincter

Stimulates penile erection

Stimulates emission (ejaculation)

Sympathetic neurons

Preganglionic   Postganglionic

Parasympathetic neurons

Preganglionic   Postganglionic

FIGURE 5-15 The Nervous System. Our nervous system is made up of a sympathetic and a parasympathetic division. Most actions by one division oppose the other. For example, the sympathetic division or nervous system inhibits digestion, whereas the parasympathetic division or nervous system stimulates digestion. (Reproduced with permission from Kibble JD. *The Big Picture Physiology: Medical Course & Step 1 Review*, 2nd ed. McGraw Hill, 2020.)

This describes the parasympathetic response.

Identification of anticholinergic toxicity can be challenging because of the constellation of symptoms from different systems that may appear unrelated. But there is a mnemonic for anticholinergic toxicity that should help you when you encounter them.

Do you remember the mnemonic for anticholinergic toxicity?

Red as a beet, dry as a bone, hot as a hare, blind as a bat, mad as a hatter, full as a flask (Figure 5-16).

What does this mnemonic mean?

Patients may appear red or flushed from the vasodilation in response to increased body temperature (*"red as a beet"* and *"hot as a hare"*).

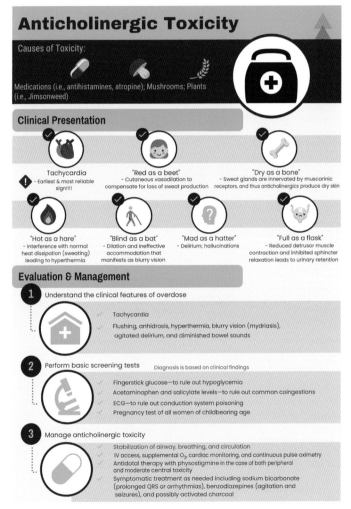

FIGURE 5-16 Anticholinergic Toxicity. The clinical presentation of anticholinergic toxicity can be remembered with the mnemonic, "red as a beet, dry as a bone, hot as a hare, blind as a bat, mad as a hatter, full as a flask." The mainstays of treatment include antidote therapy with physostigmine and symptomatic management as needed. (Reproduced with permission from Shah N. *The Infographic Guide to Medicine.* McGraw Hill, 2022.)

They may experience drying of bodily fluids, including an inability to sweat (*"dry as a bone"*).

Patient's may have decreased vision secondary to mydriasis, or pupillary dilation (*"blind as a bat"*).

In more extreme cases patients may experience central nervous system symptoms such as anxiety, agitation, confusion, or hallucinations (*"mad as a hatter"*).

Reduced detrusor muscle contraction and inhibited sphincter relaxation can lead to urinary retention (*"full as a flask"*).

If physostigmine is the correct answer, then we should see these features in the vignette.

Mannitol

Do you recall the mechanism of mannitol?

Mannitol is an osmotic diuretic.

What is mannitol primarily used for clinically?

The most common uses are for lowering of intracranial and intraocular pressure through diuresis.

In cases of increased intracranial pressure, the goal is to decrease volume inside an inflexible skull. While use of mannitol is one approach, other approaches include hyperventilation, head-of-the-bed elevation, and administration of hypertonic saline intravenously (Figure 5-17).

Insert ICP monitor—ventriculostomy versus parenchymal device

General goals: maintain ICP <20 mmHg and CPP ≥60 mmHg. For ICP >20–25 mmHg for >5 min:
1. Elevate head of the bed; midline head position
2. Drain CSF via ventriculostomy (if in place)
3. Osmotherapy—mannitol 25–100 g q4h as needed (maintain serum osmolality <320 mosmol) or hypertonic saline (30 mL, 23.4% NaCl bolus)
4. Glucocorticoids—dexamethasone 4 mg q6h for vasogenic edema from tumor, abscess (avoid glucocorticoids in head trauma, ischemic and hemorrhagic stroke)
5. Sedation (e.g., morphine, propofol, or midazolam); add neuromuscular paralysis if necessary (pt will require endotracheal intubation and mechanical ventilation at this point, if not before)
6. Hyperventilation—to PaCO$_2$ 30–35 mmHg (short-term use or skip this step)
7. Pressor therapy—phenylephrine, dopamine, or norepinephrine to maintain adequate MAP to ensure CPP ≥60 mmHg (maintain euvolemia to minimize deleterious systemic effects of pressors). May adjust target CPP in individual pts based on autoregulation status.
8. Consider second-tier therapies for refractory elevated ICP
1. Decompressive craniectomy
2. High-dose barbiturate therapy ("pentobarb coma")
3. Hypothermia to 33 °C

FIGURE 5-17 **Management of Increased Intracranial Pressure.** (Reproduced with permission from Jameson JL, Fauci AS, Kasper DL et al. *Harrison's Manual of Medicine*, 20th ed. McGraw Hill, 2020.)

Why is hyperventilation useful?

Consider the pathophysiology behind hyperventilation.

What are the physiologic changes that occur during hyperventilation?

When we hyperventilate, we are increasing the pH in the blood stream. We can remember this because hyper- refers to elevated, while hypo- refers to decreased. Thus, hyperventilation leads to an elevated pH, while hypoventilation refers to a decreased pH. Increased pH refers to a more basic environment. If the environment is more basic, then we would expect more oxygen relative to carbon dioxide. More carbon dioxide would result in a more acidic environment.

How might we expect the vasculature to change in a more basic environment with elevated oxygen and decreased carbon dioxide?

To achieve homeostasis, we would expect the vasculature to constrict. Vasodilation allows for increased oxygenation, while vasoconstriction would do the opposite. Vasoconstriction from hyperventilation will decrease intracranial pressure by decreasing the blood flow and occupied space in the skull.

Similarly, elevation of the head of the bed and administration of mannitol and/or hypertonic saline draws fluid from the intracranial space and into the systemic circulation, thereby reducing the overall volume in the skull and thus the intracranial pressure.

In the most extreme cases, a craniectomy is required to remove part of the skull to allow for more space.

In what scenario would we consider mannitol?

It would be unlikely for mannitol to be the correct answer if no imaging has been done. If we were to consider mannitol, we should have results from some diagnostic study that suggest elevated risk of, or presence of, increased intracranial pressure. Some would still not intervene with medications unless symptoms of increased intracranial pressure were present.

Even if imaging has been done, this alone is not a potent enough treatment alone for increased intracranial pressure, but rather should be used as an adjunctive treatment.

It is uncommon for adjunct treatment options to be the correct answers on standardized tests. This is the most important clue that mannitol is unlikely to be the correct answer.

Another clue is that mannitol is too vague an answer. In the case of head injury, one extreme is that the patient requires emergent surgery to relieve increased intracranial pressure, as discussed below. The other extreme is that this patient does not require any intervention at all. Somewhere in the middle lies mannitol.

Test writers prefer answers that are clearly correct and difficult to dispute. If mannitol was the correct answer, then this patient would have to have some signs or symptoms suggesting increased intracranial pressure, but not enough to warrant emergency surgery.

Emergency surgery

If there are significant clinical signs or symptoms of increased intracranial pressure or evidence of an epidural hematoma, the next best step may be an emergency craniectomy.

What are some signs or symptoms of increased intracranial pressure?

These might include nausea, vomiting, headache, visual changes, alterations in consciousness, or hemodynamic instability.

The decision for emergency surgery is highly unlikely without first obtaining CT imaging. Even with significant signs or symptoms of increased intracranial pressure, the surgeon would most likely need imaging to guide their surgical planning.

If imaging reveals an epidural hemorrhage, then emergency surgery is most likely the correct answer. With other types of hemorrhage, particularly in the absence of signs of increased intracranial pressure, emergency surgery is not necessarily the best answer.

Psychiatry consultation

Psychiatry consultation is an answer choice, like reassurance, that is often laid as a trap, but is occasionally the correct answer.

But, in the absence of other answer choices suggesting a psychiatric condition, this answer choice is less likely.

Psychiatric illnesses are challenging to diagnose in the presence of a medical condition or medication side effect(s) that might be causing or contributing to the clinical presentation. In fact, this is part of most diagnostic criteria in the *DSM-5*.

If we were to consider a psychiatric consultation, we would need to rule out other causes for mood disturbances, including metabolic derangements, toxicity, head injury, or infection.

In considering psychiatric diagnoses, acute changes in mood or mental state would be concerning for a psychotic episode. Slower, more progressive behavioral changes would be more consistent with diagnoses like anxiety or depression.

A history of psychiatric conditions could increase concern for a psychiatric etiology of her symptoms. However, the presence of a psychiatric history is more commonly a trap.

Let's summarize the diagnoses suggested by each of the answer choices. This should simplify our task of identifying the correct answer as we read the vignette.

a. *Head CT scan:* Intracranial bleed
b. *Brain MRI:* Mass
c. *Lumbar puncture:* Infection
d. *Physostigmine:* Anticholinergic toxicity
e. *Mannitol:* Increased intracranial pressure
f. *Emergency surgery:* Increased intracranial pressure
g. *Psychiatry consultation:* Mood disturbance or psychosis not caused by medical condition or medication

When we summarize the key diagnoses represented by each of the answer choices, a pattern clearly emerges; several of these answer choices are centered around intracranial pathology and increased intracranial pressure.

But is this a helpful hint, or is this a trap?

If we determine that her clinical presentation warrants further management of a head injury, then we should focus on the following answer choices:

Head CT scan, mannitol, emergency surgery, or brain MRI. This narrows our answer choices down to four.

If we decide that further management should not be focused on a head injury, then we should focus on the following answer choices:

Lumbar puncture, physostigmine, and psychiatry consultation. This narrows our answer choices down to three.

Our task will be to determine if the clinical presentation in question is from a head injury or another etiology. Based on this, we will pivot to one of the two answer choice groupings.

Just like we broke up the answer choices, you should notice that the vignette is also separated into two encounters.

What are the two encounters described in the vignette?

The patient first presents to clinic after a fall off her bicycle, and then later to the emergency department after a change in her clinical status.

You should consider the vignette in two separate parts accordingly.

Can you think of why separating these two encounters is important?

It is always important to compare how a patient was at the initial encounter from their presentation at the subsequent encounter, and what changes occurred between the encounters that may have resulted in any changes to their clinical status. Possibilities might include progression of disease processes or iatrogenic causes from interventions.

Let's read the remainder of the vignette together as though we have anchored on her head injury as the cause of all her symptoms.

The patient fell and struck her head and knee on the ground.

This describes the mechanism of injury and confirms that there was head trauma.

She did not lose consciousness.

The absence of loss of consciousness is reassuring. If there was immediate loss of consciousness, we might be more concerned about an epidural hemorrhage that would be more likely to require emergency surgery.

She subsequently developed mild nausea without emesis and head pain localized to the area of impact.

What kind of head trauma do these symptoms suggest?

While nausea, vomiting, and headache are a constellation of symptoms concerning for increased intracranial pressure, only mild nausea without emesis is more suggestive of concussion, and compared to a headache, localized pain is more suggestive of mild trauma.

Vitals and neurologic exam were normal.

Normal vital signs are reassuring, but the absence of hemodynamic instability now does not rule out the possibility later.

In the case of increased intracranial pressure, we might not expect hemodynamic instability until intracranial pressure is significantly increased and/or there is brain herniation (Figure 5-18). Other signs and symptoms will guide our suspicion for risk of clinical deterioration later.

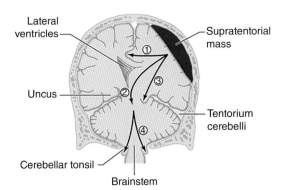

FIGURE 5-18 Types of Brain Herniation. Herniation can occur when there is mass effect that displaces brain tissue. Types include (1) cingulate herniation under the falx, (2) downward transtentorial (central) herniation, (3) uncal herniation over the edge of the tentorium, and (4) cerebellar tonsillar herniation into the foramen magnum. (Reproduced with permission from Greenberg DA, Aminoff MJ, Simon RP. *Clinical Neurology*, 11th ed. McGraw Hill, 2021.)

The patient appeared uncomfortable during the abdominal exam and scopolamine was prescribed for nausea.

The test writer is highlighting the patient's nausea. In this case, the test writer is noting that the nausea is significant enough to warrant medical intervention.

The patient presents to the emergency room the following day for agitation.

This is the subsequent encounter, and the location of her presentation is important. Initially, she presented to clinic following the injury. Now, she is presenting to the emergency room. Presentation to clinic should suggest lower acuity, while presentation to the emergency room suggests higher acuity. Higher acuity presentations are more likely to require a higher level of evaluation and/or intervention.

Her parents report that she started acting strangely a few hours earlier and has seemed increasingly agitated.

The patient has developed symptoms of altered mental status evidenced by "acting strange" and increased agitation. These symptoms were not present initially, but rather developed over the last day.

This time course decreases the likelihood of an acute hemorrhage from an epidural bleed or intraparenchymal bleed, as these bleeds tend to be fatal within several hours if not treated, though a slower bleed from a subdural hemorrhage remains a possibility. Given this information, emergent surgery is less likely the correct answer.

Medical history is only significant for allergies, which are well managed with diphenhydramine.

Medical history appears to be non-contributory. She is not presenting with allergy symptoms.

Temperature is 37.9 °C, blood pressure is 125/80 mmHg, pulse is 160/min, respirations are 22/min.

Yesterday in clinic, this patient's vital signs were normal. Today, she is mildly hypertensive and tachypneic for age with a notable tachycardia. This might be due to an underlying intracranial process.

She is pacing during the exam and is not cooperative with answering questions.

This is consistent with the parents' description of her agitation.

Pupils are equal and 7 mm bilaterally. Extraocular movements are intact.

Pupillary dilation could be concerning for brain herniation resulting in "blown pupils."

Facial movements are symmetric.

Less concerning for a focal neurologic deficit caused by a mass or ischemic event.

Mucous membranes are dry.

Perhaps due to agitation and/or increased sympathetic activation in the setting of head injury and possible intracranial pathology.

Cardiac exam is notable for tachycardia.

This is consistent with her vital signs.

Abdominal exam is notable for decreased bowel sounds and a palpable mass in the lower abdomen with mild tenderness to palpation.

We know that the patient has nausea from the head injury, which could explain the mild tenderness.

What are some explanations for the palpable mass?

There are a few possible explanations for the palpable mass.

One possibility includes internal hemorrhage secondary to trauma from the bicycle accident that was initially unnoticed or too small to detect.

Another possibility includes worsening neurological status that has resulted in an ileus with palpable stool.

Hopefully more clues will help us to determine the significance of this finding as it relates to her head injury.

The remainder of the exam is normal.

Sometimes lack of exam maneuvers mentioned in the vignette helps to narrow the differential diagnosis. If we are concerned about intracranial pathology, we might have expected the test writer to include more neurological exam maneuvers.

What information supports the hypothesis that her symptoms are secondary to head trauma?

The mechanism of injury, presence of nausea requiring medication, and head pain suggest a degree of head trauma that is not insignificant. Her worsening neurological status is concerning for intracranial process in the setting of recent head injury. Pupillary dilation and abnormal vital signs might be attributable to intracranial process and/or mass effect.

Based on this assessment, what would be the best answer choice?

As discussed earlier, a clinical presentation that is concerning for acute intracranial process such as hemorrhage requires head CT imaging as a first step in evaluation and management.

How does the time course of her presentation impact our decisions regarding best next steps?

Though her presentation to the emergency department suggests a higher acuity, the fact that this is the day after her head injury suggests that any intracranial process is subacute, not acute. This decreases the likelihood that emergent intervention is indicated.

Even with a subacute presentation, a head CT to evaluate for intracranial process seems reasonable. Though the timing is not necessarily emergent, there is no indication to suggest we need better detail from an MRI at this point.

After anchoring on her head injury as the cause of her symptoms, we were able to generate a reasonable assessment and arrive at an answer choice.

What pieces of information are we ignoring or assigning incorrect significance to by anchoring?

Recall that this vignette is divided into two encounters. There is the encounter from clinic, where her symptoms are relatively mild, and the subsequent encounter later in the emergency room, where she presents with altered mental status and vital sign abnormalities.

Let's focus first on our assessment of the initial encounter.

Our assessment of this patient after the initial encounter is reasonable. While the presence of localized head pain might be more suggestive of a skull or soft tissue contusion, the presence of nausea is more suggestive of brain trauma. Given her presentation was mild but not insignificant, a diagnosis of concussion seems reasonable. In the absence of nausea, we might only diagnose a localized and superficial injury.

For a simple concussion without concerning features, the best approach to management is supportive care without further diagnostic studies.

If we remove any anchoring bias, how would you describe her presentation in clinic?

We have a young patient who experienced head trauma from a fall off her bicycle, who subsequently developed mild nausea and abdominal tenderness, as well as localized head pain, without headache, vomiting, loss of consciousness, or focal neurological deficits.

This presentation so far is not consistent with a significant head injury warranting imaging or further intervention.

The subsequent encounter is where assumptions were inappropriately made based on "bad" anchoring.

Firstly, we labeled her behavior changes as "altered mental status." Altered mental status in the setting of head trauma is highly concerning and would typically warrant head imaging. But rather than a decreasing level of consciousness and/or neurological deficits, the patient has developed increased agitation and psychosis. These symptoms are not commonly indicative of intracranial processes, especially related to trauma.

We also attributed her dilated pupils to possible brain herniation.

If a patient has herniated, we should expect them to be obtunded or comatose. They should not be agitated and wandering around the exam room while their brain herniates.

How might we explain her abdominal symptoms in the emergency department?

Her abdominal tenderness might be consistent with her nausea that was identified the day prior. However, a palpable mass in the setting of this clinical presentation seems surprising.

While we might be able to attribute a palpable mass to constipation and/or ileus, it seems more likely that the test writer included this exam finding as an important diagnostic clue. While ileus can occur in hospitalized and/or comatose patients with decreased mobility, this patient is agitated and wandering the exam room. She is not someone we would expect to develop ileus, especially not so acutely.

Reevaluation of our initial assumptions suggests that focusing on a head injury as the underlying cause of her symptoms is incorrect.

Let's revisit the possible answer choices that were not focused on her head injury. These included *lumbar puncture, physostigmine, and psychiatry consultation.*

Is there anything that occurred between the first encounter and the second encounter that might help guide us to the correct answer?

Besides the passing of time, the only change that occurred between the first and the second encounter was the prescribing of scopolamine.

We should always pay close attention to interventions and/or medication changes that occur around the same time as symptom onset or change.

What class of medication is scopolamine?

Scopolamine is an antimuscarinic agent used for nausea. Scopolamine is probably best known for its transdermal administration over 72 hours.

Side effects are consistent with this medication's anticholinergic properties.

Given that we know she ingested an anticholinergic medication prior to the subsequent encounter to the emergency room, it is reasonable to consider physostigmine, an anticholinergic antagonist, as the correct answer.

What symptoms does she have that are consistent with anticholinergic toxicity?

As a reminder, the mnemonic for anticholinergic side effects is *red as a beet, dry as a bone, hot as a hare, blind as a bat, mad as a hatter, full as a flask.*

The patient is agitated and anxious (*"mad as a hatter"*) and has dilated pupils (*"blind as a bat"*). She is also tachycardic and mildly hypertensive, which are consistent with sympathetic nervous system activation.

How can we explain her abdominal symptoms/findings in the context of anti-cholinergic toxicity?

We know that during the "fight or flight" response, our digestive system will slow. This could explain the decreased bowel sounds. While we could still arrive at the correct answer by assuming the palpable mass is a hard ball of stool, this palpable mass is more likely a full bladder from urinary retention related to anticholinergic toxicity (*"full as a flask"*).

A distended bladder will commonly be described as a palpable mass in question stems related to anticholinergic toxicity or acute neurologic injury resulting in paralysis and urinary retention. This is a good buzz phrase to remember.

Are there any other clues that suggest anticholinergic toxicity?

During our preliminary read of the vignette, we determined that her medical history of allergies was noncontributory. This was especially true when we were anchored on the possibility of a head injury as the etiology of her symptoms.

This patient takes diphenhydramine for her allergies. Diphenhydramine, like scopolamine, has anticholinergic properties (Figure 5-19). Now that our focus is on anticholinergic toxicity, it may be easier to recognize that addition of scopolamine to her diphenhydramine regimen may have increased her risk of anticholinergic toxicity.

We should always consider the relevance of medications that the test writer chooses to include in a vignette. While the use of diphenhydramine could have been a trap, we should still take the time to consider why this was included and whether this is relevant, especially since physostigmine was one of the answer choices.

For this clinical scenario, we saw how easy it was to arrive at an answer based on generalizations and assumptions.

When we anchored on her head injury, we had to force information to fit with our mental framework.

Remember that the vignette should provide enough of support for your conclusions. If this is not the case, then it is important to rethink your conclusions.

In this case, it was important for us to examine each piece of evidence in support of our conclusion closely, rather than grouping and generalizing several findings.

Let's reread the vignette without bias or temptation to anchor and instead use evidence to support our conclusions. This will allow us to confirm whether physostigmine is indeed the correct answer, or if we are once again falling victim to anchoring.

A 10-year-old girl presents to clinic for headache following a bicycle accident that occurred a few hours earlier.

Drug Type	Strong Anticholinergic Properties
Antiemetics	Promethazine (Phenergan) Prochlorperazine (Compazine)
Antidepressants	Amitriptyline (Elavil) Desipramine (Norpramin) Doxepin (at doses >6 mg/day) Nortriptyline (Pamelor)
Antihistamines, including antivertigo medications	Chlorpheniramine (Chlor-Trimeton) Dimenhydrinate (Dramamine) Diphenhydramine (Benadryl) Hydroxyzine (Atarax) Meclizine (Antivert) Scopolamine (TransDerm Scop)
Antipsychotics	Clozapine (Clozaril) Olanzapine (Zyprexa)
Gastrointestinal antispasmodics	Dicyclomine (Bentyl)
Muscle relaxants	Cyclobenzaprine (Flexeril) Orphenadrine (Norflex)
Parkinson disease	Benztropine (Cogentin) Trihexyphenidyl (Artane)
Urinary antispasmodics	Oxybutynin (Ditropan) Tolterodine (Detrol)

FIGURE 5-19 **Anticholinergic Medications.** (Reproduced with permission from Walter LC, Chang A, Chen P et al. *Current Diagnosis & Treatment: Geriatrics*, 3rd ed. McGraw Hill, 2021.)

This sentence sets us up to focus on a head injury. The patient is presenting to clinic following the accident.

She was bicycling alongside her mother when she lost her balance as she made a turn. The patient fell and struck her head and knee on the ground. She did not lose consciousness.

Here is the mechanism for her injury. Absence of loss of consciousness is reassuring.

She subsequently developed mild nausea without emesis and head pain localized to the area of impact.

Nausea is concerning for concussion or increased intracranial pressure, but lack of emesis is reassuring. Head pain is localized only to the area of impact.

Vitals and neurologic exam were normal.

This is reassuring, though does not exclude the progression of vital sign abnormalities later.

The patient appeared uncomfortable during the abdominal exam and scopolamine was prescribed for nausea.

The patient was likely uncomfortable during the abdominal exam due to her nausea. Scopolamine was prescribed.

The patient presents to the emergency room the following day for agitation. Her parents report that she started acting strangely a few hours earlier and has seemed increasingly agitated.

She is now presenting with acute agitation that was not present yesterday. This could represent progression of an intracranial process. Alternatively, this change in her presentation might be related to the use of scopolamine given the temporal association.

Medical history is only significant for allergies, which are well managed with diphenhydramine.

Allergies do not seem significant to this presentation, but her medications do. Both scopolamine and diphenhydramine have anticholinergic properties and the combination might increase the risk of anticholinergic toxicity.

Temperature is 37.9 °C, blood pressure is 125/80 mmHg, pulse is 160/min, respirations are 22/min.

Compared to her normal vital signs yesterday, her vital signs are now abnormal.

Are there vital sign abnormalities specifically associated with increased intracranial pressure?

Cushing's triad is a concept that is infrequently tested beyond the USMLE Step 1 Exam. This triad refers to a set of signs indicative of increased intracranial pressure, and includes bradycardia, irregular respirations, and a widened pulse pressure.

While the absence of Cushing's triad does not exclude increased intracranial pressure, we could interpret this to mean there may be other possible explanations for her vital sign abnormalities.

She is pacing during the exam and is not cooperative with answering questions.

This is consistent with the parents' description of her.

Pupils are equal and 7 mm bilaterally. Extraocular movements are intact.

Pupils are dilated bilaterally, and extraocular movements are intact with an otherwise benign exam. This is less concerning for herniation or compression. Instead, we could attribute her bilateral pupillary dilation to ingestion of sympathomimetic agents.

Facial movements are symmetric.

This finding was likely mentioned to demonstrate that the patient has no focal neurologic deficits. Presence of focal neurologic deficits might indicate the need for a brain MRI.

Mucous membranes are dry.

Some possible causes could be lack of fluid intake, diabetes, or medications, particularly anticholinergic agents.

Cardiac exam is notable for tachycardia.

We know this from the vital signs.

Abdominal exam is notable for decreased bowel sounds and a palpable mass in the lower abdomen with mild tenderness to palpation.

We have discussed this finding at length already.

If we consider all the patient's symptoms together after the second encounter, then we should be able to recognize anticholinergic toxicity: Pupillary dilation, hyperthermia, tachycardia, agitation/confusion, decreased bowel motility, and urinary retention. But taken individually, arriving at diagnosis becomes more challenging, and it is easier to fall into anchoring and/or test-writer traps.

What is the correct answer?

Physostigmine

One of the most important keys to success was separating this vignette into two encounters. In doing so, the antecedent event that triggered this patient's anticholinergic toxicity becomes obvious.

SUMMARY

1. "Bad" anchoring is a bias generated from assumptions that may cloud judgment.
2. "Good" anchoring combines confidence with cognitive flexibility in response to new information.
3. We are at higher risk of ignoring or misinterpreting contradictory information when we anchor.
4. Determining whether information is useful, not useful, or a trap can protect against the dangers of anchoring.

REFERENCE

1. Olmesdahl PJ. The establishment of student needs: an important internal factor affecting course outcome. *Medical Teacher*. 1999;21(2):174–179. doi:10.1080/01421599979824.

C H A P T E R

6

Questions

QUESTION 1

A 1-year-old female is brought to the emergency department for lethargy and poor feeding. Parents noticed increased fussiness four days ago, with progressively worsening rhinorrhea and fever. She then developed emesis and diarrhea two days ago and has been refusing solids or liquids for the last 24 hours. She was previously healthy before this and takes no medications. She has a 10-year-old brother who recently recovered from similar symptoms, although the parents think his symptoms were milder. Temperature is 38 °C, blood pressure is 80/50 mmHg, pulse is 130/min, and respirations are 40/min. She is lethargic on exam. She cries without tears. Mucous membranes are dry. Cardiopulmonary exam is only notable for tachycardia and a II/VI systolic murmur. Capillary refill is 4 seconds. Dorsalis pedis pulses are 1+ bilaterally. Laboratory results are as follows:

Sodium 150 mEq/L
Potassium 3.7 mEq/L
Chloride 105 mEq/L
Bicarbonate 10 mEq/L
BUN 30 mg/dL
Creatinine 1 mg/dL

Initial management with which of the following is the next best step?

a. 0.45% normal saline
b. 0.9% normal saline
c. Intravenous ceftriaxone
d. Inhaled oseltamivir

What is a concise summary of this clinical scenario?

A 1-year-old girl is brought to the emergency department for lethargy and poor feeding for the last 24 hours in the setting of recent upper respiratory illness that started four days ago with a positive sick contact.

What is her physical exam notable for?

Lethargy and evidence of dehydration.

What are her vital signs notable for?

Fever, tachycardia, and hypotension.

What diagnoses do her vital signs suggest?

Dehydration or sepsis (Figure 6-1).

What are her labs notable for?

Elevated sodium, creatinine, BUN, and BUN/Cr ratio, with a decreased bicarbonate.

How do we interpret these labs?

Elevated sodium is likely related to her dehydration given her clinical history.

An elevated BUN/Cr ratio is suggestive of pre-renal kidney injury, likely related to her dehydration and/or likely sepsis.

•SIRS • Temperature >38 °C or <36 °C • Heart rate >90 beats/min • Respiratory rate >20 breaths/min or PCO2 <32 mmHg • WBC >12 × 10^9/L or <2 × 10^9/L or >10% immature forms
•Sepsis • SIRS + identified or suspected infection
•Severe Sepsis • Sepsis + dysfunction of one or more organ systems
•Septic Shock • Sepsis + hypotension (BP <90 mmHg or a reduction of >40 mmHg from baseline in the absence of other causes) despite adequate fluid resuscitation and perfusion abnormalities (e.g., lactic acidosis, oliguria, altered mental status)
•MODS • No current definitions

FIGURE 6-1 **Systemic Inflammatory Response Syndrome (SIRS) and Sepsis.**
(Reproduced with permission from Grippi MA, Elias JA, Fishman JA et al. *Fishman's Pulmonary Diseases and Disorders*, 5th ed. McGraw Hill, 2015.)

What is her acid-base status?

Her decreased bicarbonate is concerning for metabolic acidosis. If we calculate her anion gap, we will find that she has an anion gap metabolic acidosis. Given the clinical history, this is likely a lactic acidosis in the setting of illness and dehydration. Because she has not eaten in 24 hours, there may also be an element of ketoacidosis (Figure 6-2).

How do we categorize the answer choices?

The first three answer choices refer to fluids, whereas the last two answer choices refer to medical management for either a bacterial or influenza infection.

To answer the vignette question, we need to determine her most urgent problem.

Is her most urgent problem her fluid status or her infection?

This question is challenging because there are several pieces of information that suggest a possible meningitis and/or sepsis, in which case we would want to consider starting IV antibiotics urgently.

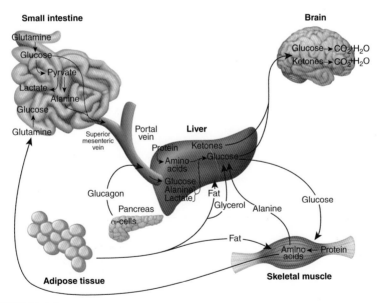

FIGURE 6-2 **Ketosis During Fasting State.** During fasting, the pancreas stimulates gluconeogenesis and glycogenolysis from the liver and fatty acid release from adipose tissue. Fatty acids may undergo oxidation in the liver to provide energy for gluconeogenesis and to produce ketones. Ketones are necessary to provide the brain with energy during periods where glucose availability is limited. (Reproduced with permission from the medical biochemistry page, LLC.)

However, there is indisputable evidence that this patient is moderately to severely dehydrated. Regardless of the underlying etiology of her clinical presentation, initiating fluids is likely the better answer.

Whether her tachycardia and hypotension are from dehydration or sepsis, fluids are first line to address her vital sign instability.

Based on advice detailed in this text, we should have been suspicious that the answer is 0.9% normal saline before even reading the vignette.

Why should we be suspicious that the answer is 0.9% normal saline?

In my experience, this is almost always the correct answer on a standardized test.

What about the other fluid choices (Figure 6-3)?

While 3%, or hypertonic, saline is not uncommon, use of 0.45%, or hypotonic, saline is exceptionally rare, especially on board exams. This answer choice may be tempting because the patient is hypernatremic. However, we know she is hypernatremic because of dehydration. Once her dehydration is corrected, the sodium should also correct.

What is the correct answer?

Normal saline

Fluid	Osmolality	Electrolytes	Indications	Precautions
D5W	Hypotonic	None	Fluid maintenance; euvolemia	Impaired glucose control in DM
0.45% NaCl (½ NS)	Hypotonic	Na+ 77mEq/L Cl– 77mEq/L	Fluid maintenance; euvolemia	Hyponatremia with long-term use; ↑ risk IV infiltration vs isotonic
0.9% NaCl (NS)	Isotonic	Na+ 154mEq/L Cl– 154mEq/L	Fluid replacement; hypovolemia, shock	Monitor for fluid overload; hyperchloremic metabolic acidosis with rapid ↑ volume
Lactated Ringer's (LR)	Isotonic	Na+ 130mEq/L Cl– 109mEq/L Lactate 28mEq/L K+ 4mEq/L Ca++ 3mEq/L	Fluid replacement; hypovolemia	Lactate converted to bicarb (liver) → alkalosis; lactate may accumulate in cirrhosis → lactic acidosis
3% NaCl	Hypertonic	Na+ 513mEq/L Cl– 513mEq/L	Severe symptomatic hyponatremia	Osmotic demyelination syndrome with too-rapid correction

FIGURE 6-3 Common IV Fluids. (Reproduced with permission from Attridge RL, Miller ML, Moote R, Ryan L. *Internal Medicine: A Guide to Clinical Therapeutics.* McGraw Hill, 2013.)

Question 1 Test-Taking Weaknesses

Anchoring
This question is designed to highlight signs and symptoms suggestive of sepsis. Anchoring on infectious symptoms could cause you to ignore the clues related to her dehydration. If you did anchor on her infectious symptoms, the answer choices related to fluid management should serve as a checkpoint to reevaluate your reasoning.

Reasoning
One of the best forms of protection against anchoring for this vignette is your ability to reason. This vignette requires you to reason through physical exam, vital sign, and lab abnormalities using your knowledge of pathophysiology.

Without proper reasoning skills, any of the abnormalities may cause you to misunderstand the vignette, second guess yourself, or anchor.

QUESTION 2

A 1-day-old boy is admitted to the neonatal intensive care unit after being born prematurely at 36 weeks as part of a twin-twin gestation. He had regular prenatal care and no abnormalities were seen on ultrasound in utero. In the NICU, he is started on high flow nasal cannula for respiratory support but is quickly weaned to nasal cannula. He takes a diet consisting exclusively of formula through an orogastric tube, as his mother is not yet producing breast milk. On day 2 of life, his oxygen requirements increase, and he becomes more lethargic. His vitals are taken, which show a temperature of 36 °C, heart rate of 200/min, and respiratory rate of 40/min. Physical exam shows a lethargic neonate with abdominal distention (Figure 6-4). Abdominal girth today is 5 cm increased compared to yesterday. Blood cultures and urine and lumbar samples are obtained but results are pending. Stool test is positive for occult blood. What is the next best step?

a. Intubate
b. Chest X-ray
c. Change food to a milk protein-free formula
d. Discontinue feeds
e. Emergent surgery

What is a concise summary of this clinical scenario?

A newborn ex-36-week-old infant develops lethargy, increased oxygen requirements, tachycardia, tachypnea, hypothermia, and gastrointestinal symptoms on day 2 of life.

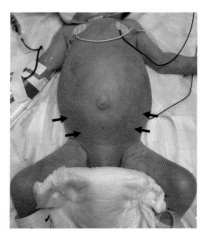

FIGURE 6-4 **Neonate with Abdominal Distension.** (Reproduced with permission from Kline MW. *Rudolph's Pediatrics*, 23rd ed. McGraw Hill, 2018.)

Let's break up this summary even further.

What is the significance of his vital sign abnormalities?

Hypothermia is more common in neonates than adults and, like hyperthermia, is concerning for infection. Concern for infection and possible sepsis is increased by his tachycardia.

Can we assume that his tachypnea and hypoxia represent a pulmonary infection?

We know that this neonate still requires oxygen support at baseline, so he may be more vulnerable to respiratory decline. Pulmonary symptoms, particularly in a neonate who is already dependent on oxygen, do not necessarily represent a respiratory infection. Respiratory symptoms might be from cardiac or respiratory failure in the setting of sepsis, or from his overall decline in mentation in the setting of lethargy. There may even be an element of respiratory compensation for a metabolic acidosis.

Are there any other abnormal systems that suggest a source for his sepsis?

There are two clues that suggest the possibility of a gastrointestinal source. The first is the mention of abdominal distention and acutely increased abdominal girth. The second is the heme positive stool.

How do we decide whether to prioritize the gastrointestinal symptoms or the respiratory symptoms?

We can consider both a respiratory and a gastrointestinal cause and decide which makes more sense based on the full clinical picture.

How would we summarize the scenario from a pulmonary perspective?

This is a preterm neonate with increasing oxygen requirements on day 2 of life in the setting of vital sign abnormalities concerning for sepsis and exam findings most notable for lethargy and tachypnea.

What are some possible etiologies for these symptoms?

Differential might include meconium aspiration (Figure 6-5), pneumonia, or respiratory distress due to lethargy in the setting of a vulnerable respiratory tract.

If this patient's symptoms were caused by a pulmonary etiology, wouldn't we expect the test writer to provide a more detailed pulmonary exam?

This could be a clue against a pulmonary etiology.

How would we summarize the scenario from a gastrointestinal perspective?

This is a preterm neonate with increasing oxygen requirements on day 2 of life in the setting of vital sign abnormalities concerning for sepsis, with acutely increasing abdominal distention and fecal occult stool testing positive for blood.

Notice how these summaries are very similar.

What are some of the key differences?

Neither perspectives acknowledge the other. Whatever perspective we ultimately choose, we need to be able to explain all the symptoms with that explanation.

Earlier, we were able to generate a reasonable conclusion about why a neonate might have respiratory failure in the setting of sepsis even without a pulmonary infection. We would be hard pressed to generate a similar conclusion to explain the gastrointestinal symptoms in the setting of an isolated pulmonary infection.

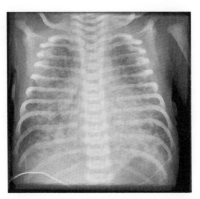

FIGURE 6-5 **Meconium Aspiration Syndrome.** Note the increased lung markings and hyperinflation. (Reproduced with permission from Gomella TL, Eyal FG, Bany-Mohammed F. *Gomella's Neonatology: Management, Procedures, On-Call Problems, Diseases, and Drugs*, 8th ed. McGraw Hill, 2020.)

Do his gastrointestinal symptoms fit with any illness script(s)?

From the perspective of illness scripts, this patient has classic risk factors and a presentation consistent with necrotizing enterocolitis (NEC). Risk factors include prematurity, formula-fed, and residence in the neonatal ICU. This alone should sway the test-taker towards a gastrointestinal source for his sepsis.

What is the ideal management for NEC?

We should discontinue feeds urgently to allow for bowel rest and obtain an abdominal X-ray to establish a diagnosis (Figure 6-6).

Is intubation a consideration?

While his respiratory status should be monitored closely, there is no indication that this patient requires intubation. While escalation of airway management is a consideration in some cases of tachypnea and increased work of breathing, there are several interventions that can be tried prior to resorting to intubation.

What is the correct answer?

Discontinue feeds

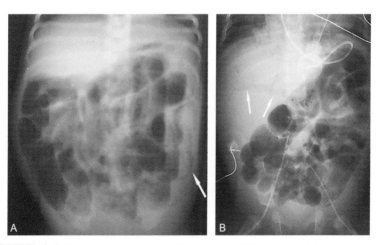

FIGURE 6-6 **Findings in Necrotizing Enterocolitis. (A)** Pneumatosis intestinalis. Abdominal X-ray demonstrates intramural gas (arrow) seen in pneumatosis intestinalis, and is a classic sign of necrotizing enterocolitis. Bowel dilation can also be seen. Portal venous gas is another classic sign of necrotizing enterocolitis, but cannot be seen on this radiograph. **(B)** Portal venous gas. Abdominal X-ray demonstrates portal venous gas (arrows) which is a classic sign of necrotizing enterocolitis. Bowel dilation can also be seen, but only minimal pneumatosis intestinalis. (Reproduced with permission from Wells RG. *Diagnostic Imaging of Infants and Children.* McGraw Hill, 2013.)

Question 2 Test-Taking Weaknesses

Anchoring

The most important strategy to prevent anchoring for questions like this is to avoid ignoring important information, like this patient's abdominal distention and bloody stool. Notice how we reasoned through both his respiratory and gastrointestinal symptoms before arriving at the best answer.

Illness scripts

This clinical presentation is textbook for necrotizing enterocolitis. Our illness script for NEC should allow us to quickly generate this diagnosis based on signs of sepsis, abdominal distension, and bloody stool, in the setting of a preterm, formula-fed neonate. Evaluation should involve abdominal X-ray +/− occult blood stool testing, and treatment involves antibiotics and bowel rest.

Remember to review concepts as illness scripts and you should hopefully remember information the same way you learned it.

Reasoning

If you were not familiar with NEC, you could still have reasoned your way to the correct answer.

After establishing that the diagnosis was related to the gastrointestinal system, we were able to exclude intubation and chest X-ray from our possible answer choices. This leaves us with the option to discontinue feeds, change to a milk-free formula, or emergent surgery. Let's think through these options.

Why isn't changing to a milk-free formula the correct answer?

We would expect isolated gastrointestinal symptoms if this was the correct answer, but this patient is also septic.

What kinds of diagnoses might be addressed with emergent surgery in our patient's case?

Given this patient has bloody stool, we might be concerned for volvulus, intussusception, or Meckel's diverticulum, but these diagnoses seem unlikely given his age and signs of sepsis (Figure 6-7). Extreme cases of NEC and/or cases refractory to treatment may also warrant emergent surgery. In our patient's case, there is nothing in the vignette to suggest the need for emergent surgical intervention.

QUESTION 3

A 28-year-old woman comes to clinic complaining of worsening dysmenorrhea. While she has always had pain associated with her menses, this pain has been

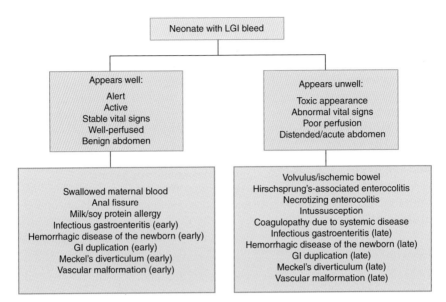

FIGURE 6-7 **Differential Diagnoses for Lower GI Bleed in a Neonate.** (Reproduced with permission from Tintinalli JE, Ma J, Yealy DM et al. *Tintinalli's Emergency Medicine: A Comprehensive Study Guide*, 9th ed. McGraw Hill, 2020.)

intensifying over the last year after discontinuing oral contraceptives. She discontinued birth control with the hope of conceiving her first child but has not yet been successful. While trying to conceive, she has also noticed worse pain with penetration during vaginal intercourse. She has never had a sexually transmitted infection and has never been pregnant. She has no medical problems and takes no medications. She does not use alcohol or tobacco products. Temperature is 37 °C, blood pressure is 110/75 mmHg, heart rate is 75/min. Patient is thin appearing. Cardiopulmonary exam is unremarkable. Abdominal exam is notable for mild tenderness in the lower quadrants. Pelvic exam is notable for some tenderness on bimanual exam with limited uterine mobility. No masses are palpated. Urine pregnancy test is negative. What is the best next step?

a. Colposcopy
b. Hormonal intrauterine device
c. Serum FSH and LH testing
d. Endometrial biopsy
e. CT scan of the pelvis
f. Laparoscopy
g. Oral contraceptives
h. No intervention is needed

What is a concise summary of this clinical scenario?

A 28-year-old woman with history of dysmenorrhea, dyspareunia, and infertility presents with worsening dysmenorrhea after discontinuation of oral contraceptives.

What is her physical exam notable for?

Mild lower abdominal and pelvic tenderness with limited uterine mobility.

What is the significance of limited uterine mobility?

This patient likely has adhesions limiting the mobility of her uterus.

What are some causes of adhesions?

Prior surgery, infection, or inflammation can cause adhesions.

What is the most likely cause of this patient's adhesions?

Given her lack of prior surgical history, combined with her history of dysmenorrhea, dyspareunia, and infertility, this patient likely has endometriosis (Figures 6-8 and 6-9).

What is the problem we need to address?

This patient is complaining of worsening dysmenorrhea ever since discontinuing oral contraceptives. We need to select an answer choice that will address her pain.

Location of Lesion	Possible Symptoms
Gastrointestinal tract	Abnormal bloating Constipation Cyclic gastrointestinal symptoms including: Diarrhea Dyschezia Menstrual catamenial rectal bleeding (rare)
Urinary tract (rarely ureteral wall)	Flank pain Hematuria (if lesion in bladder) Obstruction Urgency and frequency of urination
Pulmonary (rare)	Chest pain Cyclic hemoptysis Pleural effusion Pneumothorax/hemothorax
Brain (rare)	Catamenial headaches Seizures Subarachnoid hemorrhages

FIGURE 6-8 **Signs and Symptoms of Endometriosis.** (Reproduced with permission from O'Connell MB, Smith JA. *Women's Health Across the Lifespan: A Pharmacotherapeutic Approach*, 2nd ed. McGraw Hill, 2019. Copyright © 2019 by Mary Beth O'Connell and Judith A. Smith.)

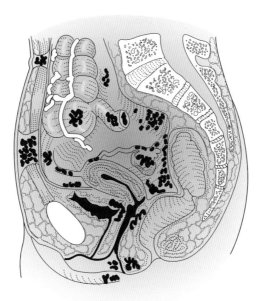

FIGURE 6-9 **Common Sites of Endometrial Implants.** Endometriosis is caused by endometrial tissue that implants outside of the uterus, referred to as endometrial implants. Endometrial tissue can implant almost anywhere in the body, but more commonly implants within the abdominopelvic cavity. Inflammation from these implants can result in adhesions. (Reproduced with permission from Way LW. *Current Surgical Diagnosis & Treatment*, 7th ed. Lange Medical Publications, 1985. Copyright © McGraw Hill.)

Are there any circumstances in this vignette that we should be mindful of when selecting a treatment option?

This patient is trying to conceive. We need to avoid any answer choices that will interfere with her ability to conceive. This point could have been missed if we read the vignette too quickly.

What is the best way to group the answer choices?

Some of the answer choices are treatment options while others are diagnostic steps.

What are the treatment option answer choices?

Hormonal IUD insertion, oral contraceptives, laparoscopy, and no intervention.

Would any of these treatment options help to reduce her pain without impacting her ability to conceive?

There are several stepwise treatment options for endometriosis (Figure 6-10).

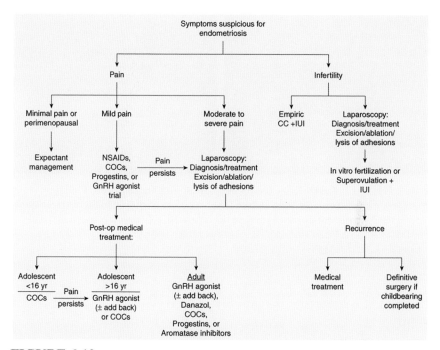

FIGURE 6-10 **Diagnostic and Treatment Algorithm for Women with Endometriosis.** (Reproduced with permission from Hoffman BL, Schorge JO, Halvorson LN et al. *Williams Gynecology*, 4th ed. McGraw Hill, 2020.)

Oral contraceptives would be a good treatment option for her pain, had she not been trying to conceive.

Laparoscopy to remove adhesions and endometrial implants could help with her pain and is also the only method to conclusively diagnose endometriosis (Figure 6-11). In fact, laparoscopy could even help with fertility.

No intervention is unlikely to be the correct answer choice because this patient both has worsening pain and an inability to conceive. We should do something.

What are the diagnostic answer choices?

Colposcopy, serum FSH and LH testing, endometrial biopsy, CT scan of the pelvis, laparoscopy, and no intervention.

As mentioned earlier, laparoscopy is the only method to definitively diagnose endometriosis and also serves as a treatment modality. If we are suspicious about endometriosis, then the remainder of these diagnostic choices would not represent the next best step.

Serum FSH and LH testing might be tempting given her infertility; however, we can assume that her infertility is likely a result of her endometriosis rather than a hormonal abnormality.

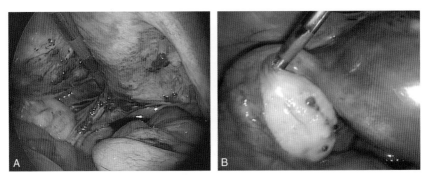

FIGURE 6-11 **Laparoscopic Images of a Patient with Endometriosis.** Findings consistent with endometriosis can be seen in these images, including bluish brown lesions seen in the posterior cul-de-sac (**A**) and on the ovary (**B**). (Used with permission from Dr. David Rogers. From Hoffman BL, Schorge JO, Halvorson LN et al. *Williams Gynecology*, 4th ed. McGraw Hill, 2020.)

On medical board exams, serum FSH and LH testing is rarely the correct answer.

CT scan of the pelvis may be considered when there is concern for malignancy, abscess, or bleed, among other uses. If you did not know the diagnosis, then you might feel tempted to pursue a CT scan.

The remaining diagnostic answer choices are classically associated with other medical problems and do not quite fit with this vignette. We know that colposcopy is done when there is concern for cervical cancer, and endometrial biopsy is done when there is concern for uterine cancer. The classic indicator for cervical cancer will be an abnormal pap smear, while the classic indicator for uterine cancer will be abnormal uterine bleeding.

What is the correct answer?

Laparoscopy

Question 3 Test-Taking Weaknesses

Categorizing information
One of the key pieces of information in this vignette is that this patient is trying to conceive. This point was mentioned in passing as the reason she discontinued oral contraceptives and it would have been easy to fail to recognize this information as important.

While we may have been able to successfully arrive at the correct diagnosis, choosing the next best step would have been difficult without acknowledging her desire to conceive. We might have focused on hormonal agents prior to considering laparoscopy.

When we practice asking ourselves why test writers choose to include certain information, we protect ourselves from missing key information like this on exam day.

Illness scripts

This vignette describes a classic presentation of endometriosis: dysmenorrhea, dyspareunia, infertility, and abdominopelvic adhesions. A solid illness script for endometriosis should make this patient easy to diagnose. But without it, these symptoms might seem vague and nonspecific.

One of the reasons these symptoms might be hard to synthesize is that many are alluded to but not explicitly stated. Her infertility is alluded in the context of her discontinuation of oral contraceptives and her uterine adhesions are alluded to with her decreased uterine mobility. Our task is to synthesize this information so that we can recognize the diagnosis and match it with our illness script(s).

QUESTION 4

A 55-year-old male comes to clinic for evaluation of a right breast mass. He first noticed a lump in his breast last week while applying sunscreen at the beach. He has no other symptoms. His medical history is notable for hypertension, but he refuses to take medications. Temperature is 37 °C, blood pressure is 147/90 mmHg, and heart rate is 85/min. Physical exam is notable for obesity and increased fatty breast tissue bilaterally. There is a 3 cm firm, fixed, nontender mass in the right breast lateral to the areola. There is no axillary lymphadenopathy. Cardiopulmonary exam is unremarkable. BMI 40 kg/m^2. What is the best next step in management?

a. Initiate blood pressure medication
b. Excision of the mass
c. Fine needle biopsy
d. Mammography
e. Serum prolactin level
f. Brain MRI

What is a concise summary of this clinical scenario?

A 55-year-old male with a history of obesity, uncontrolled hypertension, and medication noncompliance, presents for evaluation of a 3 cm, firm, fixed, non-tender breast mass.

What is the most likely diagnosis?

Given the mass is firm and fixed, his mass is more likely to be malignant (Figure 6-12).

	Benign	Indeterminate	Malignant
Shape	Oval/round	Variable	Irregular/angular, spiculations
Lobulations	Gentle bi or trilobulations	Variable	Microlobulations
Margins	Sharp/smooth	Sharp/smooth or indistinct	Indistinct/jagged
Retrotumoral acoustic phenomena	Posterior enhancement Bilateral edge shadowing	No change	Posterior shadowing, unilateral edge shadowing
Echogenicity	Hyperechoic (can also be isoechoic, anechoic, or hypoechoic)	Isoechoic or hypoechoic	Hypoechoic
Internal echo pattern	Homogenous	Variable	Heterogenous, may contain calcification echoes
Lateral-anteroposterior diameter ratio	Lateral greater than anteroposterior (ratio of lateral to anteroposterior >1)	Variable	Anteroposterior diameter greater than lateral (ratio of lateral to anteroposterior <1)
Compressibility	Compressible	Variable	Noncompressible
Compression effect on internal echoes	Echoes swirl more homogenous	Variable	No change
Adjacent architecture	Unaffected	Usually unaffected	Disrupted

FIGURE 6-12 **Features of a Benign versus a Malignant Breast Mass on Ultrasound.** (Reproduced with permission from Schrope B. *Surgical and Interventional Ultrasound.* McGraw Hill, 2014.)

What is this question testing?

This question tests your ability to identify features of a malignant mass and your knowledge of the diagnostic workup of breast cancer.

How do we diagnose breast cancer?

In terms of imaging, mammography is the gold standard for breast cancer screening and can also be used as a diagnostic tool. In younger patients, ultrasound evaluation of a suspicious mass may be a better choice over mammography given the density of breast tissue in this age group (Figure 6-13).

A core needle biopsy is the best way to evaluate a sample from the mass. This will provide enough tissue for pathologic analysis. If the mass is determined to be malignant, either lumpectomy or mastectomy will be recommended.

Are there any answer choices that suggest a diagnosis other than malignancy?

There are a few answer choices that would allow us to evaluate for gynecomastia. These include obtaining a serum prolactin level and a brain MRI.

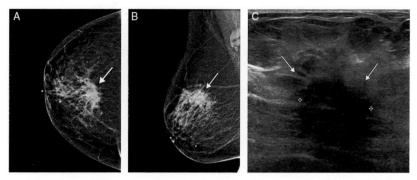

FIGURE 6-13 Breast Cancer Imaging Modalities. (A,B) Diagnostic mammograms of a large, irregular, spiculated mass (arrows). **(C)** Ultrasound image demonstrate a hypoechoic, irregular mass with posterior acoustic shadowing (arrows). (Reproduced with permission from Elsayes KM, Oldham SA. *Introduction to Diagnostic Radiology.* McGraw Hill, 2014.)

If we were concerned about gynecomastia, in the absence of any neurologic symptoms, we could start by ordering a serum prolactin level. If prolactin is elevated, a brain MRI should be considered (Figure 6-14).

Besides a prolactinoma, what are other causes of gynecomastia?

Some more common causes of gynecomastia include obesity and liver disease. This is due to the increased levels of estrogen.

How does gynecomastia classically present?

Gynecomastia should present as grossly symmetric enlargement of both male breasts and would not explain this patient's discrete, unilateral mass. All answer choices related to gynecomastia should therefore be excluded.

As we review the answer choices, we might notice that one option addresses his poorly controlled blood pressure. If we decided that this mass represented gynecomastia related to his obesity, then this might be a tempting answer choice. One clue that this is not the correct answer is that this patient has already been noncompliant with his blood pressure medications and there is nothing in the vignette to suggest he would be open to changing his mind.

What is the best next step for this patient?

We need to evaluate this patient for breast cancer. The related answer choices include excision of the mass, fine needle biopsy, and mammography.

Fine needle biopsy may be a tempting answer choice. However, a fine needle biopsy will not obtain an adequate sample for evaluation of breast cancer

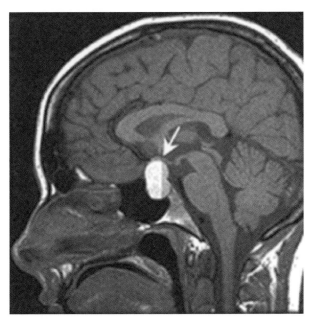

FIGURE 6-14 Magnetic Resonance Imaging of a Pituitary Adenoma. (Used with permission from Dr. Toral Patel. From Cunningham FG, Leveno KJ, Bloom SL et al. *Williams Obstetrics*, 26th ed. McGraw Hill, 2022.)

(Figure 6-15). Fine needle biopsy is commonly used for evaluation of thyroid masses, but in our case, we need a core needle biopsy (Figure 6-16).

Because core needle biopsy is not an answer choice, should we consider excision of the mass?

Rarely do we proceed with surgical intervention before obtaining imaging. We should first establish whether there is a suspicious mass on imaging and

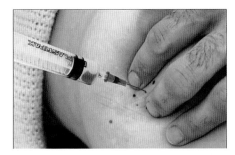

FIGURE 6-15 Fine Needle Aspiration of a Mass. Fine needle aspiration (FNA) uses a thin needle attached to a syringe to obtain small amounts of fluid and tissue from a mass. (Reproduced with permission from Barber MD, Thomas JSJ, Dixon JM. *Breast Cancer: An Atlas of Investigation and Management.* Atlas Medical Publishing Ltd, 2008.)

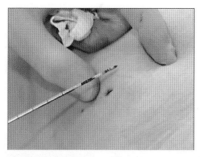

FIGURE 6-16 **Core Biopsy of a Mass.** Core biopsy uses a larger needle to remove a cylinder of tissue. Because of the use of a larger needle, more tissue can be obtained. (Reproduced with permission from Barber MD, Thomas JSJ, Dixon JM. *Breast Cancer: An Atlas of Investigation and Management.* Atlas Medical Publishing Ltd, 2008.)

whether there are any additional masses that were not palpated on exam. This will allow us to decide whether this patient may benefit from a lumpectomy or a mastectomy.

What is the correct answer?

Mammography

Question 4 Test-Taking Weaknesses

Anchoring

The patient's age and gender are not typical for breast cancer (Figure 6-17). Because of this, we could have chosen to anchor on answer choices relating to benign masses and/or gynecomastia.

The test writer also chose to include a note about his poorly controlled blood pressure. While not heavily emphasized, this is another point where we could have anchored.

Illness scripts

We should be able to easily identify concerning features of a mass, such as being fixed, irregular, or firm. And for high yield malignancies like breast cancer, we need to feel comfortable with the diagnostic work up. This is all part of the breast cancer illness script.

If we had correctly identified this mass as concerning for malignancy, the most difficult choice is likely between mammography and fine needle biopsy. If unsure, we could use our reasoning skills to arrive at the correct answer; because imaging is often pursued before invasive techniques, mammography should be a more tempting answer choice. In this case, reasoning can protect us when and if our illness scripts fail.

Age	Older
Family history	Breast cancer in parent, sibling, or child (especially bilateral or premenopausal)
Genetics	BRCA1, BRCA2, or other unknown mutations
Menstrual history	Early menarche (under age 12) Late menopause (after age 55)
Previous medical history	Endometrial cancer Proliferative forms of fibrocystic disease Cancer in other breast
Race	White
Reproductive history	Nulliparous or late first pregnancy

FIGURE 6-17 **Factors Associated with Increased Risk of Breast Cancer.** (Reproduced with permission from Papadakis MA, McPhee SJ, Rabow MW. *Current Medical Diagnosis & Treatment* 2021. McGraw Hill, 2021.)

QUESTION 5

A 38-year-old woman comes to the office for her first prenatal encounter. She has been trying to conceive with her husband for the last 5 years. She had a miscarriage 3 years ago at 15 weeks gestation and was unable to conceive a pregnancy until now. Her last menstrual period was over 8 weeks ago, and a home pregnancy test was positive. She has no other symptoms besides morning sickness. There is no history of medical conditions or sexually transmitted infections. She was drinking one to two glasses of alcohol daily before she found out she was pregnant. She does not use tobacco or illicit substances. Temperature is 37 °C, blood pressure 110/75 mmHg, heart rate 85/min. Pelvic exam is unremarkable. Bedside transvaginal ultrasound reveals a thin endometrial stripe (Figure 6-18). Urine pregnancy test done in the office is negative. Which of the following is the most likely diagnosis?

a. Early pregnancy
b. Ectopic pregnancy
c. Missed abortion
d. Incomplete abortion
e. Pseudocyesis

What is a concise summary of this clinical scenario?

A 38-year-old woman with history of infertility and miscarriage presents for evaluation after positive pregnancy test at home, without evidence of pregnancy at clinic visit today.

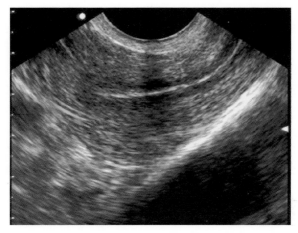

FIGURE 6-18 **Thin Endometrial Stripe on Transvaginal Ultrasound.** (Reproduced with permission from Ma OJ, Mateer JR, Reardon RF et al. *Ma and Mateer's Emergency Ultrasound*, 4th ed. McGraw Hill, 2021.)

How do we explain why there is no evidence of pregnancy in clinic today?

Because her pregnancy test today is negative, this patient is not currently pregnant. This eliminates the first two answer choices, leaving us with a missed or complete abortion or pseudocyesis.

What is pseudocyesis?

This is when a patient, particularly one who greatly desires pregnancy, is convinced that they are pregnant and may even have phantom symptoms of pregnancy.

What is the significance of her ultrasound finding?

A thin endometrial stripe suggests that there is no current intrauterine pregnancy. We already know this from her negative pregnancy test.

Would we see this finding if she was recently, but is no longer, pregnant?

If this patient was recently pregnant, we would expect to see changes to the uterine lining and cavity. Within the first few weeks, the uterine lining thickens, and a sac begins to develop (Figure 6-19). If we do not see a fetus by 6–8 weeks, but do see in-utero changes consistent with recent pregnancy, then this might suggest a recent abortion or ectopic pregnancy. But a thin endometrial stripe suggests that she has not recently been pregnant.

If there is no evidence of recent or current pregnancy, then we should presume that this is a case of pseudocyesis.

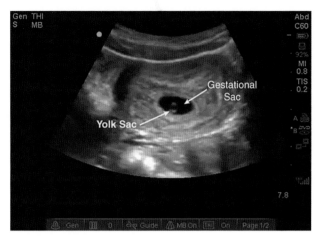

FIGURE 6-19 **Intrauterine Pregnancy Changes.** A yolk sac and a gestational sac are seen in the endometrium. (Used with permission from John P. Gullett, MD. From Shah BR, Mahajan P, Amodio J, Lucchesi M. *Atlas of Pediatric Emergency Medicine*, 3rd ed. McGraw Hill, 2019.)

What is the correct answer?

Pseudocyesis

Question 5 Test-Taking Weaknesses

Reasoning

This question is challenging for those who struggle to reason their way to an unfamiliar diagnosis.

Even if we don't have concrete knowledge about what uterine changes to expect around the time of pregnancy, we should be able to reason that there should still be visible uterine changes within a few weeks before and after a pregnancy. But, if you are unable to reason through this, there is still a good probability that you can arrive at the correct answer by reasoning through the answer choices.

The most difficult part of reasoning through these answer choices is differentiating between the types of abortions (Figure 6-20). But most of the abortion definitions are easy to figure out by their names alone.

What is a missed abortion?

If we break down the name to its literal parts, we know that an abortion was missed. We can take this to mean an abortion should have happened but didn't.

Why would an abortion need to happen?

If there was fetal demise and/or failure to develop, the body should expel the pregnancy tissue. In this case, the body has failed to do so.

Type	Internal Cervical Os	Products of Conception
Threatened	Closed	Not passed
Inevitable	Open	Not passed
Incomplete	Usually open	Partially passed
Complete	Closed	Completely passed

FIGURE 6-20 **Classification of Spontaneous Abortions.** (Reproduced with permission from Sherman SC, Weber JM, Schindlbeck MA, Patwari RG. *Clinical Emergency Medicine.* McGraw Hill, 2014.)

In the case of a missed abortion, we would expect to see evidence of a pregnancy on ultrasound.

What is an incomplete abortion?

Just as it sounds, an abortion occurs, but incompletely. This means there should be retained products of conception on ultrasound.

What is a threatened abortion?

This is when there are signs concerning for an abortion, such as bleeding and/or cramping, but no abortion has occurred yet. There is a chance that pregnancy loss will still occur.

What is an inevitable abortion?

If there is cervical dilation that cannot be treated with medical intervention, then an abortion is inevitable.

What is a complete abortion?

When the pregnancy tissue is completely expelled.

When we reason through the names, the definitions no longer seem so challenging.

Besides a complete abortion, we would expect to see some products of conception on ultrasound for each other type of abortion. This rules out missed and incomplete abortions as possible answer choices.

What about early pregnancy?

Unless this pregnancy was before her missed menstrual cycle, we should expect to see a positive pregnancy test in clinic even if it is too early to see uterine changes on ultrasound. But because this patient's last menses was 8 weeks ago, we would expect to see a positive pregnancy test and changes on ultrasound.

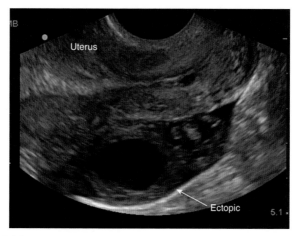

FIGURE 6-21 Ultrasound Findings in Ectopic Pregnancy. A thickened endometrial stripe is seen without an intrauterine pregnancy. An ectopic pregnancy is visible posterior to the uterus. (Used with permission from Thomas Chi, MD, FACEP. From Shah BR, Mahajan P, Amodio J, Lucchesi M. *Atlas of Pediatric Emergency Medicine*, 3rd ed. McGraw Hill, 2019.)

What about ectopic pregnancy?

An ectopic pregnancy should still produce a positive pregnancy test result. And despite not seeing products of conception within the uterus, we still might expect to see uterine changes as the uterus prepares for implantation (Figure 6-21). In the case of an ectopic pregnancy, it would be still be surprising to see a thin uterine stripe.

If we reason through the answer choices, the only possible answer choice is pseudocyesis.

We can also use our reasoning skills to guess at the definition of pseudocyesis. We know that the prefix "pseudo-" refers to something that is false or fake. If we conclude from the vignette that there has been no recent pregnancy, then it would be safe to assume that this answer choice, with the prefix "pseudo-," is most likely the correct answer.

QUESTION 6

A 10-year-old boy is brought to clinic due to 1 week of red, itchy eyes. Parents have also noticed intermittent, clear eye drainage and light crusting of both eyes when he wakes up in the morning. He has a history of mild asthma but is otherwise well. No one in the family has been sick recently but some kids at school have been sent home with rhinorrhea, cough, and pharyngitis. Temperature is 37 °C, blood pressure is 110/75 mmHg, pulse is 70/min, respirations 16/min, and oxygen saturation is 99% on room air. Physical exam is notable for bilateral conjunctival injection with mild eyelid edema. Visual acuity is 20/20 in both eyes while wearing corrective lenses. Fundoscopic exam is normal. Which of the following is the most likely cause of the patient's condition?

a. Preseptal cellulitis
b. Allergic conjunctivitis
c. Bacterial conjunctivitis
d. Viral conjunctivitis
e. Corneal abrasion

What is a concise summary of this clinical scenario?

10-year-old boy with history of asthma presents with 1 week of red, itchy eyes and clear drainage, without recent history of illness.

How do we differentiate a bacterial from a viral conjunctivitis?

A bacterial conjunctivitis should present with more severe symptoms such as pain, redness, and thick, purulent drainage that reaccumulates quickly after wiping (Figure 6-22).

Viral conjunctivitis, like allergic conjunctivitis, results in the production of thin, serous discharge and is often associated with an upper respiratory illness (Figure 6-23).

How do we differentiate a viral from an allergic conjunctivitis?

Viral and allergic conjunctivitis appear similar on physical exam, and both may co-occur with upper respiratory symptoms. In the case of allergic conjunctivitis (Figure 6-24), however, we might expect those upper respiratory symptoms to

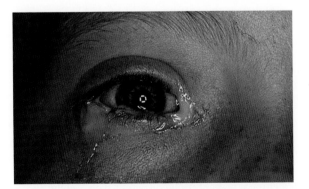

FIGURE 6-22 **Bacterial Conjunctivitis.** Bacterial conjunctivitis with mucopurulent discharge, conjunctival injection, and eyelid swelling can be seen in this image. Purulent discharge is the hallmark of bacterial conjunctivitis. (Used with permission from Frank Birinyi, MD. From Knoop KJ, Stack LB, Storrow AB, Thurman RJ. *The Atlas of Emergency Medicine*, 5th ed. McGraw Hill, 2021.)

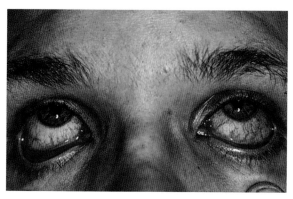

FIGURE 6-23 Viral Conjunctivitis. Viral conjunctivitis with conjunctival injection and thin, watery discharge can be seen in this image. (Used with permission from Kevin J. Knoop, MD, MS. From Knoop KJ, Stack LB, Storrow AB, Thurman RJ. *The Atlas of Emergency Medicine*, 5th ed. McGraw Hill, 2021.)

have been chronic and ongoing. The most pronounced difference is the pruritis that occurs with allergic conjunctivitis, which may result in eyelid edema from the itching and rubbing (Figure 6-24). And, while viral conjunctivitis can occur either unilaterally or bilaterally, allergic conjunctivitis should be bilateral in most cases.

What is the difference between preseptal and orbital cellulitis?

While commonly confused, recalling the difference between preseptal and orbital cellulitis is easy if you use your reasoning skills.

Preseptal refers to *before* the septum (Figure 6-25A). The septum is a fibrous layer that protects the orbit (Figure 6-26). Preseptal cellulitis will present with more superficial signs of infection involving the eyelids and proximal face.

Orbital cellulitis refers to an infection within the orbit (Figure 6-25B). Signs of orbital cellulitis, like proptosis and limited and painful eye movements, occur because of the location of inflammation within an enclosed space.

Which type of cellulitis, preseptal or orbital, is more emergent to treat?

Orbital cellulitis is an emergency, as this is a deep infection within the orbit that could compromise the eye.

Is this patient's clinical presentation consistent with a cellulitis?

In the case of this vignette, the patient is presenting with conjunctivitis as the primary problem, without any specific signs of either orbital or preseptal cellulitis. Given this, preseptal and orbital cellulitis seem unlikely.

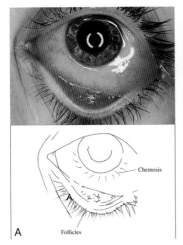
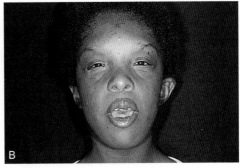

FIGURE 6-24 **Allergic Conjunctivitis. (A) Chemosis.** Allergic conjunctivitis can result in conjunctival injection and chemosis. Chemosis refers to edema of the conjunctiva from rubbing of the eyes. **(B) Eyelid swelling.** Allergic conjunctivitis with conjunctival injection, chemosis, and eyelid swelling can be seen in this image. Note mucoid discharge of both the eyes and the nose with mouth breathing. (**A:** Used with permission from Timothy D. McGuirk, DO. From Knoop KJ, Stack LB, Storrow AB, Thurman RJ. *The Atlas of Emergency Medicine*, 5th ed. McGraw Hill, 2021. **B:** Used with permission from Binita R. Shah, MD. From Shah BR, Mahajan P, Amodio J, Lucchesi M. *Atlas of Pediatric Emergency Medicine*, 3rd ed. McGraw Hill, 2019.)

How do we characterize a corneal abrasion?

A corneal abrasion refers to an abrasion of the cornea (Figure 6-27). A corneal abrasion may temporarily affect vision, though not always. The degree of conjunctival redness will depend on the degree of irritation. Itching and irritation may produce some serous discharge and eyelid swelling. This should have unilateral involvement, as it would be unusual to suffer a corneal abrasion of both eyes simultaneously.

What are some clues in his history that point to a particular diagnosis?

This patient has a history of asthma. Patients with atopic diagnoses, including asthma, allergies, or eczema, are more likely to have any of the other diagnoses. While this may be a clue, suggesting allergic conjunctivitis is the correct answer, we should also be cautious not to "bad" anchor.

This patient also has no history of recent or current illness that would suggest a viral conjunctivitis, though the absence of viral symptoms does not exclude the possibility. While the test writer notes that some children at school have had viral illnesses recently, this seems more like a trap than a helpful clue. The presence of sick contacts lacks relevance as the patient himself is not exhibiting similar signs of illness.

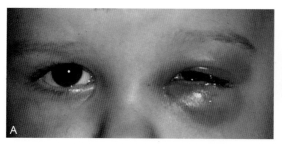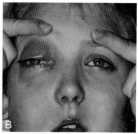

FIGURE 6-25 **Preseptal and Orbital Cellulitis.** (**A**) Preseptal Cellulitis. Patient with preseptal cellulitis. Note the periorbital swelling and redness. Occular exam itself should be entirely normal as the orbit should not be involved. (**B**) Orbital Cellulitis. Though periorbital findings are seen, like preseptal cellullitis, including swelling and redness, note the purulent drainage from the orbit and entrapment of the eye suggesting orbital involvement. (**A**: Reproduced with permission from Lueder GT. *Pediatric Practice Ophthalmology*. McGraw Hill, 2011. **B**: Used with permission from Kevin J. Knoop, MD, MS. From Knoop KJ, et al. *The Atlas of Emergency Medicine*, 5th ed. McGraw Hill, 2021.)

What are the key features from his presentation that will help us establish a diagnosis?

This patient has clear eye drainage and light crusting of both eyes when he wakes up. Clear or serous drainage suggests this is not a bacterial conjunctivitis.

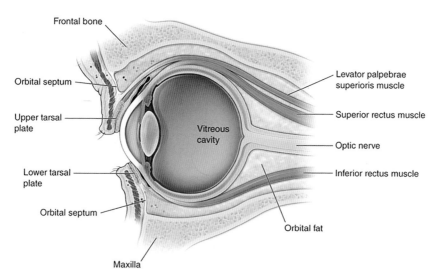

FIGURE 6-26 **Orbital Septum.** The orbital septum can be seen as an extension of the periosteum in both the upper and lower eyelids. The orbital septum acts as a physical barrier for the orbit. (Reproduced with permission from Shah BR, Mahajan P, Amodio J, Lucchesi M. *The Atlas of Pediatric Emergency Medicine*, 3rd ed. McGraw Hill, 2019.)

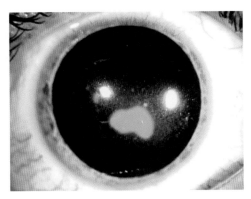

FIGURE 6-27 **Corneal Abrasion.** Fluorescein stain passes over normal cornea but will become trapped by defects. (Reproduced with permission from Kline MW. *Rudolph's Pediatrics*, 23rd ed. McGraw Hill, 2018.)

If this patient had viral conjunctivitis, we might expect continued drainage throughout the day, rather than just in the mornings.

It is highly unlikely that this patient has a corneal abrasion of both eyes, especially without a specific history that would suggest this diagnosis.

What diagnosis does his pruritis suggest?

While any conjunctivitis can cause some degree of irritation, itching is most associated with allergic conjunctivitis, especially in the absence of pain.

Why does this patient have eyelid edema?

Most likely, this edema is from itching and rubbing his eyes. The edema is mild and bilateral, without any other signs concerning for a preseptal cellulitis.

What is the correct answer?

Allergic conjunctivitis

Question 6 Test-Taking Weaknesses

Illness scripts

This question relies heavily on some knowledge about the various diagnoses. Because these diagnoses are all so similar, having established illness scripts helps to focus on the big picture, rather than getting caught up in details.

One of the key pieces of information in this vignette is the fact that this patient has itchy eyes. This is a key symptom in allergic conjunctivitis and should help to cinch the diagnosis early on.

Without illness scripts, we might have had a harder time categorizing information as useful or not useful. We may have disregarded his asthma history, or been more confused by the presence of edema, or not known the importance of bilateral versus unilateral symptoms.

Anchoring

There are a few points in this vignette where we could have been tempted to anchor.

The biggest trap in this vignette is the reference to his eyelid edema. Had we failed to identify this edema as sequelae from his itching, we might have anchored on a diagnosis of preseptal cellulitis.

If we struggle to rationalize why edema is present, we should try to set this piece of information aside rather than using it as the basis for our medical decision-making. There is enough in the vignette to contradict preseptal cellulitis that, even with the presence of edema, this is not the best answer choice.

We could have also anchored on the presence of sick contacts and clear eye drainage that could suggest viral conjunctivitis.

Oftentimes, we will see features that can fit more than one diagnosis, but we need to learn to select the choice that fits best.

QUESTION 7

A 4-year-old male is brought to the emergency department due to increasing lethargy. A few days ago, he developed a fever, myalgias, cough, and rhinorrhea. The fever was well controlled with over-the-counter medications, so his parents did not feel the need to bring him in for evaluation. His symptoms were improving until last night when he developed vomiting and lethargy. His parents brought him into the emergency department today because now he is not responding to voice and is refusing to eat or drink. His past medical history is significant for asthma, which is well controlled with albuterol as needed. He discontinued his steroid inhaler 4 months ago due to good symptom control. Temperature is 37 °C, blood pressure is 100/70 mmHg, pulse is 120/min, and respirations are 18/min. On exam, he is a lethargic appearing male who responds inconsistently to verbal stimuli. Fundoscopic exam reveals bilateral papilledema (Figure 6-28).

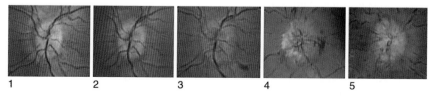

1   2   3   4   5

FIGURE 6-28 Papilledema on Fundoscopic Exam. Modified Frisén grading of papilledema, with increasing severity from left to right. Note the blurred disc margins and pale optic cup, as well as obscuration of the vasculature. (Reproduced with permission from Martin TJ, Corbett JJ. *Practical Neuroophthalmology*. McGraw Hill, 2013.)

Mucous membranes are dry. Cardiopulmonary exam is unremarkable. Abdominal exam is notable for hepatomegaly. Which of the following represent the most likely etiology for this patient's altered mental status?

a. Uremia
b. Dehydration
c. Hypoglycemia
d. Adrenal insufficiency
e. Hyperammonemia
f. Cerebral infection

What is a concise summary of this clinical scenario?

A 4-year-old male presents to the emergency department with vomiting, lethargy, and altered mental status in the setting of an upper respiratory illness.

What is the significance of his exam findings?

This patient is presenting with bilateral papilledema in the setting of altered mental status. This is highly concerning for increased intracranial pressure.

His abdominal exam is notable for hepatomegaly. Whatever is causing his altered mental status should also explain his hepatomegaly.

What is the significance of his vitals?

His vital signs are notable for a normal temperature of 37 °C, a normal blood pressure for age of 100/70 mmHg, and a normal heart rate for age of 120/min.

These normal vitals suggest against infection or sepsis that might be contributing to his worsening presentation. Given this, it is unlikely that an intracranial infection is causing his altered mental status or increased intracranial pressure.

How might hepatomegaly co-occur with altered mental status?

If this patient's hepatomegaly was suggestive of liver failure, then we might become concerned for hyperammonemia. If ammonia levels become elevated enough, then patients can become encephalopathic. This could explain both the liver and neurologic symptoms.

Are there any reasons why this patient might have acute liver failure?

If we reread the vignette, the only precipitating factors for his acute clinical change were his febrile upper respiratory infection and the over-the-counter antipyretics that were given for his fever. We should think through whether these precipitating factors might result in liver failure.

How might these precipitating factors result in his clinical presentation?

We need to come up with a diagnosis that explains this patient's whole clinical picture. It is hard to think of a virus that can cause upper respiratory symptoms, hepatomegaly, neurologic symptoms, and vomiting. While CMV or EBV are common viral illnesses associated with hepatomegaly, they are not typically associated with liver failure (Figure 6-29). And while viral hepatitis might result in vomiting, liver failure, and encephalopathy as a result, it would be incredibly unlikely for this patient to have a concurrent upper respiratory illness and a viral hepatitis.

If an infectious etiology can't explain all of his symptoms, then we should consider whether any anti-pyretic medications might result in liver failure.

The most tested medication that results in liver failure is acetaminophen. But acetaminophen is not likely to result in liver failure unless overdosed and/ or taken concurrently with alcohol. We would only expect an overdose for a patient in this age group if there was a case of accidental ingestion.

Are there any other antipyretic medications that could explain his encephalopathy and hepatomegaly?

Aspirin is associated with an increased risk of developing Reye syndrome.

What is Reye syndrome?

Reye syndrome is a disorder involving encephalopathy and hepatic dysfunction that results following a viral illness.

Signs and Symptoms	Percent of Subjects		
	EBV (Age 14–35 Years)[a]	EBV (Age 40–72 Years)[b]	CMV (Age 30–70 Years)[c]
Fever	95	94	85
Pharyngitis	95	46	15
Lymphadenopathy	98	49	24
Hepatomegaly	23	42	N/A
Splenomegaly	65	33	3
Jaundice	8	27	24

FIGURE 6-29 **Comparing EBV with CMV.** (Reproduced with permission from Kaushansky K, Prchal JT, Burns LJ et al. *Williams Hematology*, 10th ed. McGraw Hill, 2021. [a]Data from Hoagland RJ. *Am J Med Sci.* 1960;240:21. [b]Data from Hoagland RJ. *Am J Med Sci.* 1960;240:21; Schmader KE et al. *Rev Infect Dis.* 1989;11:64; Axelrod P, Finestone AJ. *Am Fam Physician.* 1990;42:1599; and Hurwitz CA et al. *Medicine (Baltimore).* 1983;62:256. [c]Data from Just-Nubling G et al. *Infection.* 2003;31:318; and Cohen JI, Corey GR. *Medicine (Baltimore).* 1985;64:100.)

If you were not able to recall details about Reye syndrome, remember that you don't need this information to answer this question correctly. We just need to identify that liver failure is present and could explain his encephalopathy.

Could uremia explain his encephalopathy?

While uremia could result in encephalopathy, there is no obvious mechanism to explain why he would have become uremic. And this would not explain his hepatomegaly.

What is the significance of his recent discontinuation of his steroid inhaler?

This information alludes to the possibility of adrenal insufficiency, but this is a trap. It is highly unlikely if not impossible for prolonged steroid inhaler use to result in adrenal insufficiency.

What is the correct answer?

Hyperammonemia

Question 7 Test-Taking Weaknesses

Categorizing Information

Whenever a test writer includes recent medication changes, we need to evaluate whether this is useful, not useful, or a trap. In the case of the antipyretic medication usage, this was useful information that led us to the correct answer. But in the case of the steroid inhaler, this was a trap as well as an opportunity to "bad" anchor.

Illness Scripts

If we do not have an illness script for meningitis, we might feel tempted to select this as the answer. We could reason a way in which an upper respiratory infection resulted in meningitis causing his neurological changes. However, not only would this ignore his liver involvement, but fails to consider the overall clinical picture.

If we have built an illness script for Reye syndrome already, this clinical scenario should be easy to identify right away. The keys here are: *recent upper respiratory illness, use of over-the-counter medications, encephalopathy, and liver failure.* Our ability to identify scenarios like this quickly will allow us to work efficiently and effectively.

QUESTION 8

A 25-year-old African American male comes to clinic due to excessive urination. He first noticed this a few months ago after starting a new job as an airline pilot. He has found that he needs to void every few hours during the day and his co-pilot has started to make comments about his urinary frequency. He is uncomfortable with this attention and is worried he will be fired from his job. In addition, he is more tired at work lately, which he attributes to waking in the middle of the night to void. He has tried to restrict his fluids to 1 L daily, but this has not resulted in a significant change. He denies any pain with urination, urethral discharge, or pain with ejaculation or defecation. His medical history is only notable for obsessive-compulsive disorder, which has been well controlled on clomipramine. He takes no other medications. Family history is significant for a mother who died at age 52 from chronic kidney disease related to her diabetic nephropathy and a father who died at age 40 from sickle cell disease. Vital signs and physical exam are entirely unremarkable. Urinalysis reveals the following:

Specific gravity: 1.00
pH 6.0
Protein negative
Blood negative
Glucose negative
Ketones negative
Leukocyte esterase negative
Nitrites negative

What is the most likely cause for this patient's polyuria?

   a. Primary polydipsia
   b. Hyposthenuria
   c. Conversion disorder
   d. Factitious disorder
   e. Medication side effect
   f. Diabetes mellitus
   g. Diabetes insipidus

What is a concise summary of this clinical scenario?

A 25-year-old male airline pilot with a history of obsessive-compulsive disorder presents with new urinary frequency without dysuria or urethral discharge.

What are clues from his history that might suggest one diagnosis over another?

We learn that this patient has a notable family history of chronic kidney disease from diabetic nephropathy as well as sickle cell disease. It is not common for test writers to include such specific family history, and so we should take the time to consider whether there is any relevance to the vignette.

The test writer also hints at psychiatric themes at several points throughout the vignette. They highlight his worry about losing his job, his increased tiredness, and his history of obsessive-compulsive disorder, for which he takes clomipramine. If we review the answer choices, we can see that a few are psychiatric diagnoses as well as the option of a side effect from his psychiatric medication causing his symptoms. We need to determine whether the psychiatric references are useful or a trap.

What answer choices should be considered if we are leaning towards a psychiatric diagnosis?

Primary polydipsia, conversion disorder, and factitious disorder.

In this case, the test writer notes that the patient restricts fluid without noticing a difference in symptoms. This suggests against the diagnosis of primary polydipsia.

This patient is unlikely to have factitious disorder as he does not stand to benefit from his excessive urination, and in fact, seems distressed by these symptoms.

Conversion disorder is typically a diagnosis of exclusion related to neurologic symptoms and does not seem like a plausible explanation for this patient's symptoms.

Would clomipramine explain this patient's presentation?

Clomipramine is a tricyclic antidepressant with anticholinergic properties.

How might anticholinergic medications effect the urinary system?

Recall the mnemonic discussed earlier in the text for side effects of anticholinergic medications: "*red as a beet, dry as a bone, blind as a bat, mad as a hatter, hot as a hare, full as a flask.*"

"*Full as a flask*" refers to urinary retention that can be a side effect of anticholinergic medications. With urinary retention, we may see overflow incontinence resulting in more frequent urination of small volumes.

Does this fit with the clinical history in the vignette?

While this patient is having increased frequency, there is no mention of incontinence or small volumes of urine with voiding. Additionally, urinary retention with overflow incontinence would not explain his decreased specific gravity on urinalysis (Figure 6-30).

Going back to his family history, is this information useful or is it a trap?

Let's first consider his mother's history of chronic kidney disease from diabetic nephropathy. His mother's kidney disease was caused by diabetes, which this patient has no history of, rather than an inheritable, primary renal disease.

Let's now consider his father's history of sickle cell disease (Figure 6-31). This patient has no medical history of sickle cell disease but could be a carrier.

Type of Urinary Incontinence Description

Functional	Includes people who have normal urine control but are unwilling (impaired cognition) or who have difficulty reaching a toilet in time because of muscle or joint dysfunction or environmental barriers
Stress	Describes the loss of urine during activities that increase intra-abdominal pressure such as coughing, lifting, or laughing. Stress incontinence is also particularly noted in high-impact sports that involve running and jumping, gymnastics, and basketball
Overflow	The constant leaking of urine from a bladder that is full but unable to empty due to • anatomic obstruction, for example, prostate enlargement • neurogenic bladder, for example, spinal cord injury
Urge	The sudden unexpected urge to urinate and the uncontrolled loss of urine; often related to reduced bladder capacity, detrusor instability, or hypersensitive bladder

FIGURE 6-30 Types of Urinary Incontinence. (Reproduced with permission from Dutton M. *Dutton's Orthopaedic Examination, Evaluation, and Intervention*, 5th ed. McGraw Hill, 2020.)

Are there any medical problems that arise from being a sickle cell carrier?

Most people with sickle cell trait live their entire lives without medical problems. However, there are some that will have decreased urinary concentrating abilities, known as hyposthenuria, and may even be at increased risk of renal disease.

Are there any clues in the vignette that suggest hyposthenuria?

This patient has a low specific gravity.

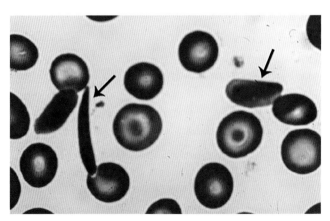

FIGURE 6-31 Sickled Red Blood Cells under Microscope. (Reproduced with permission from Lichtman MA, Shafer MS, Felgar RE, Wang N. *Lichtman's Atlas of Hematology*, 2nd ed. McGraw Hill, 2017.)

What is the relevance of a low specific gravity?

Specific gravity is a measure of urinary concentration. High specific gravity suggests a highly concentrated urine, whereas a low specific gravity suggests impaired concentration ability. In our patient's case, his urinalysis demonstrates poor concentrating ability.

Diabetes insipidus could explain his poor urine concentrating abilities and is a very tempting answer choice. However, we need to consider the whole picture and the clues laid out by the test writer. There are no clear triggers, such as recent head injury, that might suggest a new presentation of diabetes insipidus. The only recent change was starting his new job as an airline pilot, which requires him to spend more time in high altitude conditions.

How could high altitude explain his symptoms?

Increased altitude has a number of effects on the body, one of which is increasing urinary frequency. While this can be a physiologic process that occurs in all individuals, a patient with hyposthenuria might notice these effects more.

What is the correct answer?

Hyposthenuria

Question 8 Test-Taking Weaknesses

Reasoning

If you did not know the definition of hyposthenuria, then you might need to rely on reasoning to arrive at the correct answer choice.

We can reason through the word to arrive at the definition, or at least get closer to it. We know that *hypo-* refers to less, and we know that *-uria* refers to urination. While we can't necessarily reason our way to the precise definition, we could reason enough to conclude that this most likely represents a decreased ability to concentrate urine. This would explain the only abnormality on his urinalysis.

Anchoring

This vignette hints at psychiatric features throughout the vignette, ultimately highlighting this patient's use of clomipramine. Clomipramine is commonly associated with urinary side effects. If we did not take the time to think through the specific urinary side effects we see with tricyclics, we might feel tempted to anchor on medication side effect as the correct answer. Or, we might feel tempted to select one of the other psychiatric diagnoses as our answer.

By now, we should feel well prepared to resist premature anchoring and test-writer traps.

QUESTION 9

A 45-year-old female comes to clinic for evaluation of thigh pain. She first noticed a "pins and needles" sensation with associated numbness over the lateral aspect of her right thigh 2 months ago after starting a new job as a flight attendant. She feels that her thigh pain and numbness are worse when she is at work. This job is more physically demanding compared to her last job as a receptionist, though she does not recall any specific injury or precipitating event. She changed jobs over the last year after a manic episode resulted in the loss of her job, but she reports her mood has been stable after starting olanzapine. Past medical history is notable for bipolar disorder I. Vital signs are unremarkable. BMI is 39 kg/m^2. On examination, the patient is an obese female in no acute distress with normal affect. There is an area of numbness and burning pain over the anterolateral thigh extending from just below the hip to just above the patella. Straight leg raise is negative bilaterally. Strength is 5/5 bilaterally and reflexes are intact. Which of the following is the most likely cause of the patient's symptoms?

a. Meralgia paresthetica
b. Herniated disc
c. Varicella Zoster
d. Medication side effect
e. Factitious disorder
f. Diabetic neuropathy

What is a concise summary of this clinical scenario?

A 45-year-old woman, with medical history only notable for bipolar disorder I and obesity, presents with neuropathic pain and numbness over the anterolateral thigh, worse after starting a job as a flight attendant, without any known precipitating injury.

Lets consider how the location of her symptoms helps us to narrow the diagnosis.

If this patient had diabetic neuropathy, what kind of distribution might we expect?

Diabetic neuropathy most commonly effects the hands and feet in a peripheral and bilateral distribution. Neuropathic symptoms only involving the unilateral thigh would be surprising.

If this patient had varicella zoster, or shingles, what kind of distribution might we expect?

While we typically associate varicella zoster with skin findings, neuropathic pain can occur prior to the vesicular skin eruption. However, varicella zoster virus follows a dermatomal distribution and does not cross midline (Figures 6-32 and 6-33). While our patient's rash may not cross midline, the extension across

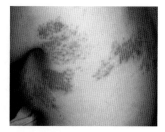

FIGURE 6-32 **Herpes Zoster Rash.** Classic shingles rash in the T4 dermatome. (Reproduced with permission from Kang S, Amagai M, Bruckner AL et al. *Fitzpatrick's Dermatology*, 9th ed. McGraw Hill, 2019.)

the length of the anterolateral thigh crosses more than one dermatome, making varicella zoster unlikely.

If this patient had a herniated disc, what kind of distribution might we expect?

A herniated disc, like varicella zoster, should follow a dermatomal distribution (Figure 6-34). Unlike varicella zoster, however, a herniated disc should produce

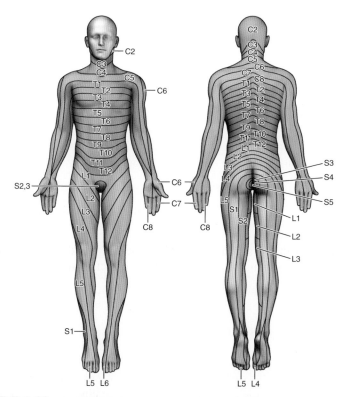

FIGURE 6-33 **Dermatome Map.** (Reproduced with permission from Diwan S, Staats PS. *Atlas of Pain Medicine Procedures.* McGraw Hill, 2015.)

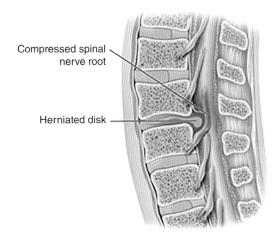

FIGURE 6-34 **Herniated Disc.** Herniated disc compression of the spinal nerve root. (Reproduced with permission from Parks E. *Practical Office Orthopedics*. McGraw Hill, 2018.)

weakness in addition to sensory symptoms. This is because there is compression of the entire nerve root.

If this patient had peripheral neuropathy of a single nerve, what kind of distribution might we expect?

Peripheral nerves do not usually follow dermatomal distributions as they are often composed of nerves from multiple nerve roots. Peripheral nerves may be sensory, motor, or both.

We now have a better sense of the pathophysiology behind her symptomatology and have been able to rule out some answer choices.

If we review the remaining answer choices, we see that we have to determine whether her neuropathic symptoms are from a medication side effect, factitious disorder, or meralgia paresthetica. We have already ruled out varicella zoster, herniated disc, and diabetic neuropathy based on the distribution of her symptoms.

There is a lot of additional information about this patient's social and behavioral circumstances included in the vignette. We should determine whether this information is useful, not useful, or a trap.

How can we summarize this additional information?

This patient with a history of bipolar disorder I recently started a new job as a flight attendant since losing her job after a manic episode at work. This is when her symptoms started. Her bipolar disorder is now well controlled on olanzapine.

The test writer also highlights her obesity twice. This emphasis suggests that this information is more likely to be useful than to be not useful or a trap.

Why is the test writer highlighting her obesity?

While you do not need to understand this point to answer the question correctly, the test writer is likely alluding to the fact that she has gained weight recently after starting olanzapine, and subsequently started a new job as a flight attendant where she might be wearing a tight-fitting uniform, and now has neuropathic symptoms.

Based on the timing of events, we can hypothesize that her symptoms are from compression of a nerve from the uniform, with obesity as a risk factor.

Her job as a flight attendant could have served as a trap for some test-takers. If we had misunderstood the vignette, we might have felt tempted to consider that her new job, which requires her to be more active, resulted in a herniated disc. But this would be an incorrect conclusion.

What is the significance of her psychiatric history?

One of our tasks as the test-taker is to determine whether her symptoms are directly related to the initiation of olanzapine.

What are the most common symptoms from olanzapine?

Olanzapine, like other second-generation antipsychotics, carries a risk of weight gain and metabolic disorders. Neuropathy should not be a side effect of this medication.

Her psychiatric history also serves as a trap to lure test-takers to select factitious disorder as their answer, but there is nothing to support this answer choice. A psychiatric history alone is not enough to conclude factitious disorder is the cause of her symptoms.

While we may not recognize meralgia paresthetica, deductive reasoning will still allow us to arrive at this correct answer. The suffix "algia" refers to pain and paresthesia refers to a neuropathic skin sensation. Taken together, we can conclude that this condition involves pain and neuropathic sensations of the skin, in this case of her thigh.

Meralgia paresthetica is a condition caused by compression of the lateral femoral cutaneous nerve where the nerve passes underneath the inguinal ligament (Figures 6-35 and 6-36). This is a purely sensory nerve, so we don't expect to see weakness. Risk factors for nerve compression include tight clothing, obesity, and pregnancy.

What is the correct answer?

Meralgia paraesthetica

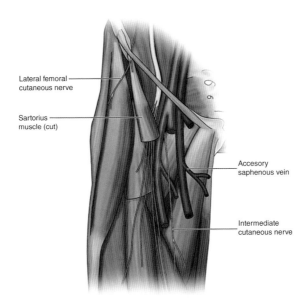

FIGURE 6-35 **Lateral Femoral Cutaneous Nerve Passing Underneath the Inguinal Ligament.** (Reproduced with permission from Diwan S, Staats PS. *Atlas of Pain Medicine Procedures*. McGraw Hill, 2015.)

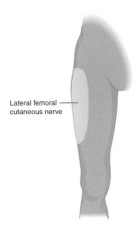

FIGURE 6-36 **Sensory Distribution of the Lateral Femoral Cutaneous Nerve.** (Reproduced with permission from Greenberg DA, Aminoff MJ, Simon RP. *Clinical Neurology*, 11th ed. McGraw Hill, 2021.)

Question 9 Test-Taking Weaknesses

Reasoning

This question preys on test-takers that suffer from underconfidence. Our best weapon in this case is our reasoning skills.

We did not need to know anything about meralgia paresthetica to answer this question correctly. With a solid understanding of the pathophysiology of the peripheral nervous system and neuropathies, we are still able to arrive at the correct answer.

Categorizing Information

There is a lot of information contained within this vignette that might seem difficult to assign meaning to. For example, many test-takers may not understand the relevance of the social circumstances detailed by the test writer. While this extra information is helpful, it is not necessary to arrive at the correct answer.

When we don't know whether information is useful or not useful, the best strategy is to move on. If we become anxious or insecure about our lack of knowledge, we limit our ability to overcome our weaknesses.

Anchoring

This vignette highlights a recent change to her medications after a manic episode resulting in the loss of her job. We often associate recent changes to medications and/or medical conditions to be important for arriving at the correct answer. But we always need to be cautious and note when this is a trap.

In this case, the test writer spent much of the vignette detailing her social circumstances, which might further tempt the test-taker to anchor on a psychiatric diagnosis like factitious disorder or a medication side effect as the cause of her symptoms. This is intentional by the test writer.

When we anchor, we fall into the temptation of selecting an answer because it seems right even without much support. We can avoid anchoring by remembering to have specific, good reasons why an answer is supported or not supported.

QUESTION 10

A 66-year-old man is brought to the emergency department due to cough and fever. He has had a chronic cough for the last year that has worsened over the last 3 days. Yesterday, he began having chills and measured a temperature of 38 °C at home. His daughter insisted he come to the emergency department today for evaluation. Medical history is significant for hyperlipidemia and diabetes mellitus of 20 years. He has also had recurrent pneumonia infections over the last 6 months. He is a former smoker of 20-pack-years. Temperature is 38.5 °C, blood pressure 110/70 mmHg, and pulse 100/min. On exam, there is decreased air movement in the right upper lobe with rhonchi at the base. Cardiac exam is normal. There is no lower extremity edema. X-ray reveals a consolidation in the right upper lobe and he is started on amoxicillin-clavulanate (Figure 6-37). Laboratory results are as follows:

Serum sodium: 115 mEq/L
Serum potassium: 3.7 mEq/L
Serum creatinine 0.9 mg/dL
Serum osmolality 260 mOsm/kg
Urine osmolality 700 mOsm/kg

What is most likely to reveal the cause of the patient's electrolyte abnormalities?

a. Chest CT
b. Brain MRI
c. Renal biopsy
d. Serum cortisol
e. Desmopressin stimulation test

What is a concise summary of this clinical scenario?

A 60-year-old man, who has a 20-pack-year smoking history, hyperlipidemia, diabetes, and recent recurrent pneumonias, presents with signs and symptoms concerning for pneumonia, found to be hyponatremic.

What are we trying to determine as the test-taker?

While most of the vignette is focused on pulmonary symptoms, our focus should be on determining the cause of his electrolyte abnormalities.

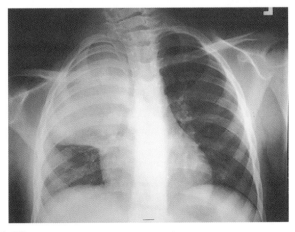

FIGURE 6-37 Right Upper Lobe Pneumonia. A lobar consolidation can be seen in the right upper lobe on this chest radiograph. (Used with permission from Binita R. Shah, MD. From Shah BR, Mahajan P, Amodio J, Lucchesi M. *Atlas of Pediatric Emergency Medicine*, 3rd ed. McGraw Hill, 2019.).

Is his pulmonary illness relevant to his electrolyte abnormalities?

When we see electrolyte abnormalities combined with pulmonary illness, we should always think of SIADH. This is a pattern, or illness script, that is very high yield. Many pulmonary processes can result in SIADH, but SIADH is associated most commonly with small cell lung cancer on exams.

What evidence do we have to suggest this patient has SIADH?

Our first step in determining whether this patient might have SIADH is to evaluate the labs.

As a reminder, the labs are as follows:

Serum sodium: 115 mEq/L
Serum potassium: 3.7 mEq/L
Serum creatinine 0.9 mg/dL
Serum osmolality 260 mOsm/kg
Urine osmolality 700 mOsm/kg

How would you interpret these labs?

This patient is significantly hyponatremic with a low serum osmolality and a borderline elevated urine osmolality. His potassium and creatinine are roughly normal.

We know that hyponatremia can occur with excessive fluid reabsorption, as seen in SIADH, and with excessive fluid loss, as seen in diabetes.

What is the best way to distinguish between the two?

The best way to distinguish between the two is to compare the serum to the urine osmolality. In this case, we have a low serum osmolality and a high urine osmolality. This suggests excess fluid retention and is consistent with SIADH.

What is the mechanism of SIADH?

Recall that excessive ADH is secreted in SIADH, resulting in excess fluid reabsorption at the expense of sodium balance. SIADH is considered a euvolemic hyponatremia because the body can regulate volume with aldosterone but is unable to regulate sodium levels due to the inappropriate ADH secretion.

Why might this patient have SIADH?

We discussed that many pulmonary processes can result in SIADH, but that SIADH is most commonly associated with small cell lung cancer on exams.

Are there any clues in the vignette that suggest a lung pathology other than pneumonia?

The test writer notes that this patient has a recent history of acute onset recurrent pneumonias.

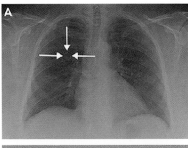
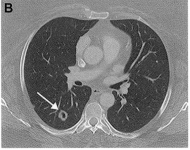

FIGURE 6-38 **Adenocarcinoma of the Lung.** A: Chest X-ray demonstrates a round lesion in the right upper lung field. B: Chest CT demonstrates a walled cavitary lesion, with adenocarcinoma confirmed on biopsy. (Reproduced with permission from Elsayes KM, Oldham SA. *Introduction to Diagnostic Radiology.* McGraw Hill, 2014.)

What might predispose this patient to recurrent pneumonias?

This presentation in a patient with significant smoking history should be concerning for an obstructive mass that is predisposing to recurrent infections. This, combined with probable SIADH, is highly concerning for malignancy.

Because we suspect pulmonary malignancy is causing his SIADH, a chest CT is most likely to reveal the cause of this patient's electrolyte abnormalities (Figure 6-38).

What are the goals of the test writer for this question?

The test writer wants the test-taker to both diagnose SIADH and to identify the risk factor that this patient has for developing SIADH. Only then can the test-taker arrive at the correct answer.

What is the correct answer?

Chest CT

Question 10 Test-Taking Weaknesses

Reasoning

If we were struggling to arrive at the correct answer, we could have employed our reasoning skills.

The first step would be to reason through his electrolyte abnormalities.

The key finding in this vignette is his low sodium and serum osmolality with a relatively high urine osmolality.

From a basic understanding of osmolality, we can recognize that the serum is diluted whereas the urine is concentrated. From this, we can deduce that there is a problem with his ADH regulation. We know that the problem is ADH because we know that ADH regulates sodium concentration through free water uptake. By thinking through this pathophysiology, we are not tempted to worry about a cortisol problem, which the test writers have hinted at with the borderline low potassium.

The next step is to consider why he might have SIADH and what studies would reveal this etiology. If we have no idea why, we can think through the answer choices.

As a reminder, the answer choices are as follows:

a. *Chest CT*
b. *Brain MRI*
c. *Renal biopsy*
d. *Serum cortisol*
e. *Desmopressin stimulation test*

Would a desmopressin stimulation test reveal the etiology of his SIADH?

A desmopressin stimulation test can be used to differentiate between central and nephrogenic diabetes insipidus. We might have selected this answer choice if we had confused diabetes insipidus with SIADH.

The remaining answer choices include chest CT, brain MRI, and renal biopsy.

A renal biopsy seems like an unlikely choice before conducting any further testing. At this point, we don't have a good reason to suspect renal pathology and would not jump to an invasive procedure yet.

A brain MRI could be tempting if you conclude a pituitary cause for his SIADH. One argument against a brain tumor is that this vignette was focused on pulmonary symptoms. On the other hand, if we are thinking like a strategic test-taker, then we might conclude that the test writer is trying to lure us towards a pulmonary etiology, when really this patient requires a brain MRI for a pituitary tumor.

The big question is: what is useful, and what is a trap?

Though test writers can be tricky, they need to provide enough support in the vignette to answer the question. A brain tumor in this patient would seem farfetched without any other relevant backstory.

The best supported answer in this case is a chest CT.

Categorizing Information

This vignette includes a lot of information about this patient's pulmonary processes, but the key to establishing a diagnosis of malignancy is his history of recurrent pneumonias over the last 6 months. If we had not identified this information as useful, we might not have realized the need for a chest CT.

When information is heavily emphasized in a vignette, we know that this information will either be useful or a trap. It might be tempting to categorize his pulmonary processes as a trap, but reasoning through the sequence of events and pathophysiology should guide you to the correct answer choice.

Index

Note: Page numbers in **boldface** indicate a major discussion. Page numbers followed by *f* indicate figures.